AF269553

MOVEMENT OF KNOWLEDGE

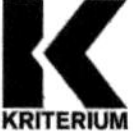
KRITERIUM

Movement of knowledge

Medical humanities perspectives on medicine, science, and experience

Edited by
Kristofer Hansson & Rachel Irwin

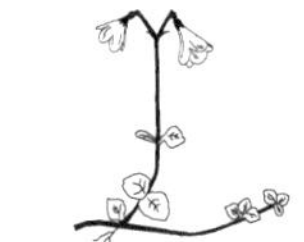

NORDIC ACADEMIC PRESS

CHECKPOINT

Nordic Academic Press
P.O. Box 148
SE-221 00 Lund
Sweden
www.nordicacademicpress.se

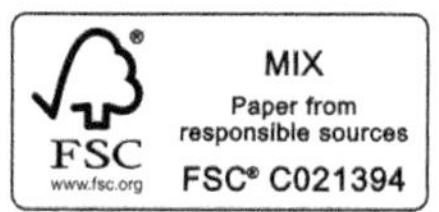

For enquiries concerning printing/copying this work
for commercial or extended use please contact the publisher.

© Nordic Academic Press and the Authors 2020

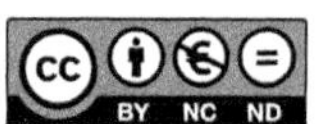

This volume is an edition from Nordic Academic Press Checkpoint – a series dedicated
to peer-reviewed books. It is also published within the framework of Kriterium, a quality
hallmark for Swedish academic books. All Kriterium publications undergo peer review
according to set guidelines, and are available as open access publications at www.kriterium.se

Translations: Charlotte Merton Gray
Typesetting: Frederic Täckström, Sweden
Cover design: Anette Rasmusson
Cover photo: Kristofer Hansson
Print: ScandBook, Falun, Sweden 2020
ISBN 978-91-88909-34-3 (print)
ISBN 978-91-88909-36-7 (epdf)
ISSN 2002-2131 Kriterium (Online)
DOI 10.21525/Kriterium.24

Contents

Preface

Knowledge about the body is constantly increasing, generating new treatments, therapies, and policies for our commonest diseases. At the same time, these are changes that create entirely new and at times revolutionary views of what it means to be human. Concerned with the social, cultural, and aesthetic factors in medical science, the medical humanities address such issues. One of its approaches is to examine how knowledge flows between different actors, whether researchers and the public, medical experts and patients, or within the global flow of knowledge in general. These are the tides and currents in which medical knowledge of individuals and communities takes shape. In this volume, humanities researchers follow the ebb and flow of knowledge between different actors and contexts, and argue for a review of modern medicine.

The volume is the product of a number of research collaborations within the Cultural Studies Group of Neuroscience at the Department of Arts and Cultural Sciences, Lund University. The group's members are involved in a number of multidisciplinary environments, and we would like to express our warmest thanks to all the research environments concerned for the opportunities for a rewarding scientific collaboration. The first is Bagadilico, a research consortium funded by the Swedish Research Council from 2008 to 2018, which conducts fundamental medical research on Parkinson's disease and Huntington's disease. The acronym Bagadilico is taken from the first two letters of each of the words Basal Ganglia Disorders Linnaeus Consortium, the basal ganglia being the part of the brain where some nerve cells die, leading to the development of these two diseases. The second is LUC3—Lund University Child-Centred Care—at Lund University, which is funded by FORTE, whose fundamental health science research looks at how health services can best support children with long-term illnesses, promoting good health for life. Our research group has also had the good fortune to collaborate with 'Falsified medicines in a multicultural society: Importance of knowledge exchange between the public and expertise' funded by the LMK Foundation, a research node that focuses on fundamental medical and pharmaceutical research into counterfeit medicines in modern society.

We would like to extend our thanks to all our research colleagues for many enthusiastic discussions. Such collaborations are what make it possible to share in the everyday life of research laboratories and clinics. There have been any number of meetings, seminars, interviews, and observations, without which our research and this volume would not have been possible. We look forward to similarly fruitful collaborations in future. We owe a great debt of thanks to the Joint Faculties of Humanities and Theology at Lund University. And finally, we wish to thank our reviewers for their careful reading of earlier drafts of this book, while singling out Daniel Normark of the Centre for Science and Technology Studies at Uppsala University and the Unit for Medical History & Heritage at the Karolinska Institutet for his kind efforts in seeing the volume to completion.

Kristofer Hansson, Malmö, 2020

Previous publications by the Cultural Studies Group of Neuroscience include *The atomized body* (edited by Susanne Lundin, Max Liljefors & Andréa Wiszmeg, 2012), *Modern genes* (Niclas Hagen, 2013), *Interpreting the brain in society* (Kristofer Hansson & Markus Idvall, 2017), a special issue of *Culture Unbound* on 'The unbound brain' (guest-edited by Peter Bengtsen & Kristofer Hansson, 2018), and *Cells in culture, cells in suspense* (Andréa Wiszmeg, 2019).

Movement of knowledge
Introducing medical humanities perspectives on medicine, science, and experience

Kristofer Hansson & Rachel Irwin

Medical knowledge is always in motion. It moves from the lab to the office, from a press release to a patient, from an academic journal to a civil servant's desk and then on to a policymaker. Knowledge is deconstructed, reconstructed, and transformed as it moves. The dynamic, ever-evolving nature of medical knowledge has given rise to different concepts to explain it: diffusion, translation, circulation, transit, co-production. At the same time, its movements—and the ways in which we conceptualize and describe them—have material consequences. For instance, value judgements on the validity of certain forms of knowledge determine the direction of clinical research. Policy decisions are taken in relation to existing knowledge. The acceptance or rejection of treatment protocols based on medical 'facts' impacts patients, dependents, health providers, and society at large. Simply put, knowledge and the movement of knowledge matter.

How do they matter, though? The contributors to this volume examine the complexity of medical knowledge in everyday life. We demonstrate not only the pervasive influence of knowledge in medical and public health settings, but also the range of methodological and theoretical tools to study knowledge. Ours is a multidisciplinary approach to the medical humanities, presenting both contemporary and historical perspectives in order to explore the borderlands between expertise and common knowledge. The medical humanities have a long history of addressing questions of context, experience, and representation in medical and public health settings (Cole et al. 2015), and thus have an enduring interest in the relationships, and expectations of these relationships, among the various actors who have a part in the motion of knowledge, whether medical specialists, policymakers, or, of course, patients and their carers.

Many of the chapters have an empirical basis in southern Sweden. The research has been carried out in close collaboration with medical researchers, practitioners, and patients, and thus reflects a specific form of healthcare setting which is strongly influenced not only by the 'traditional' Swedish welfare model, but also by the neoliberalization of this model in recent decades (see also Nordgren & Hansson 2019). In this way, our research can be framed as something that Peter Keating and Alberto Cambrosio (2006) define as a biomedical platform, or a set of activities where biomedical research, meetings between professionals and patients, the communication of medical information, and so forth take place. Such a platform 'is more than an instrument or device, but is a specific configuration of instruments and individuals that share common routines and activities, held together by standard reagents' (23). One of our themes is how medical knowledge is part of common routines and activities, and we also consider how these kinds of platforms influence and are influenced by the configurations of globalization and neoliberalization. The discourses and practices of clinical trials, diagnostics, and policymaking take similar forms wherever one is in the global scientific community, yet at the same time we see how these processes are situated in specific local contexts. In this way, the volume contributes not only to the development of medical humanities perspectives in Sweden, but is also relevant to international scholars.

Each of the chapters highlights the need to reflect on the movement of knowledge and to create a bridge between different disciplines, thus widening the opportunities for the humanities and sciences to collaborate. Medical knowledge influences everyday life, both in medical settings and beyond. We argue that an interdisciplinary approach will not only improve the handling of clinical encounters, but will also improve everyday life outside the clinic (Mol 2008). In this introduction we look at how medical knowledge can be addressed in the medical humanities vis-à-vis the main empirical themes of the volume. The wide range of approaches is a reflection of the multifaceted nature of the concepts used to describe the movement of knowledge. This is further evident as we present the chapters, which provide a breadth of perspectives on medical knowledge, illuminating different aspects of the journey and offering ways forward.

Conceptualizing knowledge

The medical humanities have a role in the continuously evolving world of biomedicine, for mediating and scrutinizing the new and unstable knowledge produced in different arenas. In this volume, we borrow the concept of multistability from the post-phenomenologist and philosopher of science Don Ihde (2012), which, when applied to knowledge, acknowledges that it is used by different actors for different purposes, and that it has different and multiple meanings in different periods and contexts. This becomes apparent in the study of medical knowledge in contemporary healthcare and biomedicine.

At the same time, the concept of multistability must be contextualized, for there is a long research tradition in both the humanities and the social sciences of focusing on questions concerning the nature and production of knowledge (Pickstone 2000). For instance, society entered a post-industrial era in the 1950s and 1960s, characterized by growing health and education sectors—and a transformation of how knowledge was valued and handled (Drucker 1969; Bell 1973). This is explored in Anna Tunlid's chapter on how prenatal diagnosis changed not only the production of knowledge in medical research, but also public debate: new medical knowledge from the rapidly expanding biomedical research field resulted in new views on the prenatal body.

In the late 1970s and 1980s postmodernism came to dominate all kinds of solid knowledge, instead arguing that there were no longer any knowledge values that were superior to others (Lyotard 1979). The postmodern theory of knowledge posited by social constructionism also provides a starting point for critiquing the relationship between knowledge and power. In the humanities this perspective has had a significant influence on both research methods and theories, not least in the medical humanities. In fact, this change has been fundamental to the medical humanities as a field, and all the chapters in this volume relate to social constructionism to some degree.

This intimate relationship between knowledge and power is also found in the work of Michel Foucault (1980), one of the most influential researchers in the field of medical humanities. For instance, the chapters in this volume address how knowledge is controlled and used to control, while at the same time influencing power structures—that is, knowledge bases are used to justify courses of action (Gutting 2005). This is writ large in healthcare settings, where a body of evidence can promote certain policies over others. Kristofer Hansson's chapter, for example, focuses on how technology and medical knowledge in diabetes care are used to justify certain actions, and how technology and knowledge mediate relationships between the families of children who have been diagnosed with diabetes and health professionals.

Others have focused on authoritative knowledge. What counts or does not count as knowledge is a long-standing concern in the social sciences, science and technology studies (STS), anthropology, and sociology. Many scholars have critiqued biomedicine as an unquestioned and now dominant cultural system (see Latour & Woolgar 1979; Mishler 1981; Starr 1982; Jordan 1983; Hahn & Gaines 1985). Using Sheila Jasanoff's term 'co-production' (2004) we would argue that knowledge is not only socially and culturally produced, but that it also generates the sociocultural context in which researchers are situated. Jasanoff defines scientific knowledge as something that 'both embeds and is embedded in social practices, identities, norms, conventions, discourses, instruments and institutions' (2004, 3). Several of the chapters in this volume expand upon Jasanoff's co-production concept, and similarly we argue that there is a need for a focus on the myriad connections between all the actors in the biomedical platform. The individual chapters provide examples of this co-production, but it is when we take a view of the whole platform that a broader analysis is possible. We cannot separate knowledge from the lifeworld in which we live (Husserl 1972), which means that knowledge is closely linked to and depends on power and culture, science, medicine, and society. The philosopher Ian Hacking (1996) discusses looping effects: how knowledge not only gives us new perspectives on life, but also changes actual life practices. In medicine, new categorizations—for example, a new way of measuring or defining disease—also means that we as researchers, medical professionals, and patients act in new ways. The anthropologists Margaret Lock and Mark Nichter (2002) pursue this idea by drawing on Foucauldian motifs to describe the export of biomedicine as a form of governmentality and neo-colonialism. They write that the processes of modernization and Westernization have imposed norms for 'what counts as evidence, legitimacy in policymaking, privileged knowledge, definition of disease categories' (3–4, 10), which in turn causes tensions 'between traditional values that define identity and the forces of modernization and globalization' (8) and fuels a debate about the dominance of a specific paradigm, evidence-based medicine.

Knowledge and evidence-based medicine

It is through the lenses of power, knowledge, and authority that specific developments in evidence-based medicine have been described. We use evidence-based medicine as an umbrella term to describe developments—over roughly the past thirty years—in how knowledge is validated, and the use of 'robust' testing to produce knowledge. Evidence-based medicine is often defined as 'the process of systematically finding, appraising, and using contemporaneous research findings as the basis for clinical decisions' (Roberts & Yeager 2006, 68; see also Rosenberg & Donald 1995), and we analyse it from a variety of theoretical and empirical perspectives. Originating from medical science, evidence-based medicine is considered first-rate knowledge with ostensibly objective verifications of reality, and as such is the kind of methodologically robust knowledge that medical professionals and biomedical researchers value. At the same time, this knowledge, when it is circulated and shared, is juxtaposed with practical relevance (Bohlin & Sager 2011), as discussed in Rachel Irwin's chapter here. Medical knowledge does not always reflect the lived experience of health professionals, patients, and carers.

The push for evidence-based medicine in healthcare from the turn of the twenty-first century has radically changed the medical care offered to patients, as well as changing the work environment in hospitals and laboratories (see also Bohlin & Sager 2011; Berner & Kruse 2013). This same perspective on knowledge is finding its way out from healthcare, something that is addressed in Karolina Lindh's chapter on the role of press releases about the latest science discoveries in how knowledge produced in laboratories reaches the public.

A closely connected development is the ongoing digitalization of life, which is transforming how we relate to and process evidence-based knowledge. New digital tools are an important part of the development of contemporary biomedical research and medical practice (Beaulieu 2004; Dumit 2004; Carusi & Hoel 2014). Digital patient registers, digital monitoring, digital diagnostic tools, and other technologies change the ways nurses and doctors work, and, in a broader sense, healthcare has been reorganized to accommodate evidence-based medicine about the patient and the patient's body. It is crucial in both hospitals and laboratories 'that we can talk about a new form of medicine—informatics medicine—with its own practices of knowledge and development' (Eklöf & Normark 2018, 345). At the same time, this informatics medicine offers important social arenas and global markets in which patients and others can discover new knowledge and treatments that are not offered by their local healthcare systems.

From a medical humanities perspective, we see major advantages in revisiting classic studies to gain new perspectives on the latest developments in medicine. The study of evidence-based medicine with the concept of authoritative knowledge was developed by the medical anthropologist Brigitte Jordan in her study, *Birth in Four Cultures* from 1978 (1993), in which she demonstrates how technology created a 'regime of power' in the birth process by generating authoritative knowledge and delegitimizing indigenous knowledge about the birth process. Authoritative knowledge is 'the knowledge that is constructed and displayed by members of a community of practice as the basis for legitimate decision-making' (xiii). In any given domain, parallel knowledge systems exist, but one often gains primacy (150–1). Authoritative knowledge emerges as the 'natural' way of things, even though it is a cultural system that is consciously and unconsciously reproduced. In this framework, some kinds of knowledge count and others do not, regardless of 'truth value' (149). In the example of birth and reproduction, Jordan finds that doctors often rely on technology (such as foetal heart monitors) rather than the mother's experience or the experience of (non-professional) midwives. In a contemporary perspective, evidence-based medicine can be said to be a form of authoritative knowledge, as discussed here in Rui Liu and Susanne Lundin's chapter on the grey market in medicines and how different knowledge regimes challenge one another. We would argue that a key methodological perspective in the medical humanities is to understand evidence-based medicine relative to what can be called everyday experience.

Knowledge in everyday experience

Everyday experience provides a starting point when questioning traditional doctor–patient relationships or patients' and carers' lived experiences, both of which are crucial to understanding the movement of knowledge and whose knowledge 'counts' (Frykman &

Gilje 2003; Normark 2019). The span is wide. They can be patients with Parkinson's disease understanding informed consent in a medical trial, as in Markus Idvall's chapter; they can be parents whose children have recently been diagnosed with diabetes and are trying to understand care practices, as in Hansson's chapter. In terms of phenomenology, a focus on the knowledge created from everyday experience provides insight into what it means to be human in varying medical practices (Becker 1992; King et al. 2017). In this vein, the philosopher Julia Kristeva and her colleagues have invited us to rethink the medical humanities:

> A new programme for the medical humanities should involve a radical concern with cultural dimensions of health as more than a subjective dimension outside the realm of medical science. We will explore the notion that *all* clinical encounters should be considered as cultural encounters in the sense that they involve translation between health as a biomedical phenomenon and healing as lived experience. Hence, our assumption is that the cultural crossings of care are not an exception but the norm. Given this, every clinical encounter should involve a simultaneous interrogation of the patient's and the doctor's co-construction of new and shared meanings that can create realities with medical consequences, not 'mere' symbols of 'real' medical issues. (Kristeva et al. 2018, 57)

Much of the focus of the present volume is the public reconstruction of knowledge from medicine and science (Rose 2007; Gottweis 2008; Hansson 2017). It can be a person sitting at a computer trying to understand online knowledge; a patient meeting a doctor or nurse; a member of the public reading a press release about a new medicine; a person sitting in front of a piece of art as in Max Liljefors's chapter. It is from such a perspective that some of the multistability of knowledge can be understood. Taking a more philosophic perspective, it becomes clear that the question is centuries old. Ludwig Wittgenstein's admission 'I don't merely have the visual impression of a tree: I *know* that it is a tree' (*On Certainty,*

§267) is central, but when do we *know*? In this volume we are not interested in what can be defined as truth and knowledge per se; instead, our methods are designed to gauge the lifeworlds of those who interpret the knowledge that surrounds them.

Borrowing from the historian James A. Secord (2004), we discuss knowledge in transit. Secord's proposed change in perspective on knowledge has been central for humanities research in recent years (Östling et al. 2020), and we find the move away from knowledge as a communicative action to knowledge as a form of doing of science to be a fruitful one. Specifically, Secord writes that 'we need to shift our focus and think about knowledge-making itself as a form of communicative action' (2004: 661), and in discussing knowledge in transit he argues that knowledge should always be seen as a form of communication. Indeed, the communicative aspects of knowledge are increasingly central considerations in medicine, healthcare, and public health.

We offer examples of the communicative aspect to science transmission between researchers, between researchers and the public, and between civil servants and policymakers. Such practices are central not only to any understanding of how science and medicine produce knowledge, but also to how knowledge production is a form of knowledge in action (see Schütz & Parsons 1978). For instance, as medical knowledge circulates it is also enacted. This enactment consists of what people do with 'information artefacts'—how press releases, articles, and books are not only embedded in a context, but also are used in different ways (Buckland 2012), as examined in Åsa Alftberg's and Lindh's chapters. For the medical humanities, a central question is therefore how knowledge from biomedicine and healthcare is set in motion in the everyday lives of patients or relatives (Kleinman 1988).

The relationship 'between health as a biomedical phenomenon and healing as lived experience' (Kristeva et al. 2018, 57) is not unproblematic. Modern medicine has long viewed biomedical phenomena as 'largely free from values, meaning and desire, as opposed to the afflicted laypeople's views' (Wiszmeg 2017, 74). This begs the question of which actors have the best arguments: Is it the researchers or the public? Is it the medical doctors or the patients (Wynne 1996; Pellizzoni 2001)? Recent years have seen a change, as the contradictions between science and alternative facts, especially in the social media, are exposed, which is considered here in Liu and Lundin's chapter about falsified medicines. Digitalization has led to the spread of knowledge and is a platform for creating and resolving differences of opinion. For example, we find communities of so-called fact resisters who are seemingly impervious to facts that contradict their own perception. This has given rise to movements that rally to the defence of medical knowledge and its significance for a modern, progressive society (see Frans 2017), which may involve practitioners where, for example, advocates of alternative approaches argue that vaccination programmes are risky, invoking alternative information in social media. Communication is also often discussed in relation to the questioning of evidence-based medicine by, for example, the anti-vaccination movement.

While it is important to defend medical knowledge, in the humanities we are interested in understanding the various actors' perspectives rather than criticizing them (see also Haraway 1985; Latour 2003; Rose 2013; Hansson & Lindh 2018; see also Hansson, Nilsson & Tiberg in this volume). While fact resistance and online discussions may lead to illegalities—such as purchasing counterfeit medicines online as Liu and Lundin describe in this volume—they also highlight what is missing in society. As Lindh asks in her chapter, what happens when evidence and popular understanding, politics and ideology, conflict? From a medical humanities perspective, we argue that studying differences of opinion or the lack of trust in biomedicine offers key insights into the ways in which medical knowledge moves.

Presentation of the chapters

The volume falls into four sections, each addressing a specific issue of how medical knowledge relates to biomedical platforms. It begins with a section—'Medical knowledge and the political'—that focuses on the biomedical platform as part of a sociopolitical context, investigating relations between communities and healthcare systems, and with medical knowledge seen as something that moves between them, affecting political decisions which, in turn, affect the healthcare system. The next section—'Circulating and sharing medical knowledge'—focuses on how medical knowledge circulates in biomedical platforms and how researchers share knowledge with other researchers or the public. The third section—'Co-creation of medical knowledge'—focuses on the ethical tools and co-creation of evidence-based medicine as a way to bridge between the posited circulation of 'objectified' knowledge and therapeutic knowledge. Finally, section four—'Knowledge in everyday experience'— develops therapeutic knowledge and its interface with patient and patient families with a focus on self-knowledge.

The first section starts with Anna Tunlid's chapter, 'Prenatal diagnosis: Co-production of knowledge and values in medical research and public debate', a discussion of how social, political, and ethical factors formed an integral part of foetal diagnostics when they were developed and used in a clinical context in the 1960s and 1970s, as well as how these factors affected the public debate about foetal diagnosis in the early 1980s. Informed by Jasanoff's conclusions about co-production (2004), Tunlid analyses the interplay between the development of knowledge and societal norms and values. The purpose is to show how medical knowledge of chromosomes, syndromes and disabilities was embedded in norms, values, and practitioners, and how the perception of foetal diagnosis was affected. This included everything from how healthcare practitioners should inform parents about foetal diagnosis to views on abortion. The medical knowledge and practical technology (foetal diagnostics) were interpreted differently in different social contexts. A dominant view in medicine is that cultural, social, and political values are barriers to be overcome; however, given co-production, Tunlid demonstrates that these values are integral to how biomedical technology, such as foetal diagnostics, is applied and regulated in society.

Regulation is also the topic of 'Evidence-informed policymaking at the World Health Organization', in which Rachel Irwin looks at how knowledge, evidence, and experience are used in the WHO's policymaking process. She compares two WHO recommendations—the UNICEF/WHO International Code of Marketing of Breastmilk Substitutes from 1981 and the Set of Recommendations on the Marketing of Foods and Non-alcoholic Beverages to Children from 2010—using interviews with key stakeholders, participant observation at the WHO's headquarters in Geneva, Switzerland, and archival material. As the UN's specialized agency for health, the process of drafting recommendations considers systematic reviews of scientific literature, recommendations set by expert committees, and data on disease trends and burdens. At the same time, the WHO is a political organization, and major policies must be agreed by all 194 member states who, in turn, are influenced by a range of private sector and civil society actors. Irwin examines how knowledge—in the form of evidence and experience—is used in the policy process, demonstrating with extended, historical case studies the changes in the type and quality of evidence used in policymaking, the different standards applied to determine what counts as knowledge, and the challenges of setting policy in the absence of evidence and experience.

In the second section—'Circulating and sharing medical knowledge'—the contributors' empirical base is modern biomedical settings, for example laboratories or communication professionals who translate the latest discoveries into press releases. Åsa Alftberg's chapter 'Sharing knowledge: Neuroscience and the circulation of knowledge', uses neuroscientists' reflections on how they share knowledge and findings, and especially the challenges, opportunities, and ethical dilemmas, to examine the knowledge circulation of cutting-edge neuroscience. A central topic is how scientific knowledge is sometimes seen as personal property that can be problematic to share with other researchers, but on other occasions sharing can be seen as something positive, with multiple career benefits for the individual researcher or for a research group. By examining the view that knowledge and knowledge circulation are the preserve of a privileged group—the creators of knowledge—Alftberg highlights the complexities of knowledge circulation. She also discusses how and why knowledge circulates, and what happens when knowledge ceases to be the exclusive property of a particular group and is used and transformed by other groups.

This perspective on circulation is further elaborated on by Karolina Lindh in the chapter 'Press releases as medical knowledge: Making news and identification in medical research communication'. Medical knowledge about the brain is not confined to labs, clinics, or the neuroscientific community. One way in which such knowledge leaves the labs and scientific communities and reaches the public is in the form of press releases. This chapter contributes with understandings about the negotiations that occur in the practices of writing these press releases. Press releases are understood here as a genre that facilitates social action. This implies that those involved in creating press releases must have a shared understanding of how press releases are written and read, and how the readers make sense of them. The chapter is based on interviews with communication professionals and neuroscience scholars working at two different Swedish universities. In this empirical material, Lindh examines the negotiations between different actors that occur as medical knowledge is transformed into press releases.

In the third section—'Co-creation of medical knowledge'— action is considered to be something that is co-created. Markus Idvall examines informed consent procedures in clinical trials for Parkinson's disease treatment in 'The co-production of informed consent: How mutual trust is negotiated between scientists and participants in clinical trials'. Using ethnographic fieldwork at a university hospital, including observations, focus-group discussions, and interviews with doctors, nurses, patients with Parkinson's disease, and their carers, he looks at the knowledge process which the informed consent procedure triggers between scientists and participants. Drawing on Jasanoff (2004), he uses the concept of co-production to describe the process as informed trust, rather than informed consent. Specifically, he demonstrates how this process is not limited to the actual signing of an informed consent document, but rather how trust is negotiated—and renegotiated—between the patient and scientists before, during, and after the trials. These relations build on the interplay of the scientists' expert knowledge and the embodied experience of patients and their carers and their lay knowledge, as scientists and patients exchange sets of knowledge in the course of the trials. There are expectations on both sides. A 'good' research subject is a knowledgeable one, who takes responsibility; the responsibilities of the scientist include sharing information about the trial and the state of research on Parkinson's. However, the fragility of the consent process is undeniable.

Various processes of co-production and co-creation are also addressed in 'The co-creation of situated knowledge: Facilitating the implementation of care models in hospital-based home care' by Kristofer Hansson, Gabriella Nilsson, and Irén Tiberg. They argue that the evidence-based care models introduced into healthcare are a form of ontology that calls for specific ways of treating concepts such as healthcare, patient, treatment, and care. Such models aim to create a certain kind of explanation of a complicated reality where they are intended to work, but often there are so-called epistemological breaks, as a result of which the models are perceived incorrectly, create the opposite effect, or have unintentional consequences. These epistemological breaks are manifest during the implementation of new care models, when evidence-based medicine meets the older knowledge contained in the healthcare professionals' existing practices, habits, and performances. The chapter sets out an ethnographic method that can be used during such implementation processes to help bring together evidence-based care models and older knowledge as new care practices. The method focuses on how best to support the facilitator of the implementation of the group when they have to address any epistemological breaks that may arise; as the authors point out, knowledge is something that all involved must work on actively throughout the implementation process, truly creating situated knowledge together, and understanding that these different knowledges are the way forward.

The last section—'Knowledge in everyday experience'—continues with the healthcare context with Kristofer Hansson's chapter 'A Number in Circulation: HbA1c as standardized practice in diabetes care'. HbA1c is a blood value that measures how much sugar is bound to the red blood cells—haemoglobin (Hb)—which, since the red blood cells are broken down after about 120 days and newly formed, can be used to assess the effectiveness of diabetes treatment. HbA1c readings are expressed in numbers, but these numbers are interpreted, translated, and understood in different ways depending on the context in which they are presented and used. In an ethnographic study, Hansson examines how the numbers are discussed in meetings both between health professionals and newly diagnosed children and their parents, and in working group meetings of health professionals. It is found that figures in medicine form normative guidelines, with numbers perceived as different types of knowledge depending on how they are used in practice. Specifically, the chapter considers the value 52 as a matter of knowledge—not just a figure that patients and families strive to achieve in the course of their treatment, but also a figure that generates a certain relationship between healthcare professionals and patients and their families. Similarly, it is also a figure that affects healthcare, with ramifications for quantification, measurement, and standardization in medicine.

The focus narrows to the purely individual in Max Liljefors's chapter 'Knowledge worlds apart: Aesthetic experience as an epistemological boundary object', which details a research project with an art exhibition for patients with Parkinson's disease, organized at an art gallery. Within the framework of the project, a new educational method was developed that focuses on aesthetic experience and bodily self-knowledge. This is in contrast to traditional art education, which primarily deals with art history and interpretation. In this way, Liljefors combines contemporary findings from the growing field of culture and health with older insights derived from aesthetic philosophy to argue that aesthetic experiences can constitute an essential aspect of the health dimension that is increasingly called 'existential' or 'spiritual' health. The chapter ends with an appendix where the current project method is described in detail with pedagogical texts and photographs.

In the final chapter, Rui Liu and Susanne Lundin re-evaluate traditional models of the doctor–patient relationship in 'Medicines in the grey market: A sociocultural analysis of individual agency'. They draw on survey data and netnography to chart individuals' experiences buying medicines online. Liu and Lundin argue that deregulation of the retail pharmaceutical sector in Sweden opened the way to online sales of medicines, and while many sellers are legitimate pharmacies, consumers risk purchasing medicine of unknown providence from illegal or quasi-illegal sources. They find that the doctor–patient dialogue is not a hierarchical one, and that people take in multiple forms of knowledge, not only consulting their doctor, but also friends and even strangers online, and relying on their own experience. In a health system and society with neo-liberal characteristics like Sweden, the individual is expected to take responsibility for self-care, and part of this involves gathering and synthesizing information, and making one's own treatment decisions.

*

Knowledge matters to all disciplines, including the medical humanities. Changes in biomedicine and healthcare require fresh knowledge perspectives, along with completely different ways of approaching the wider cultural and social context in which healthcare takes place. While we believe that the medical humanities have a given place in this co-construction of new knowledge, we also argue that the field needs to further develop its theories and methodologies. Our hope is that this volume will help the medical humanities to more fully address the movement of knowledge.

References

Beaulieu, Anne (2004), 'From brainbank to database: The informational turn in the study of the brain', *Studies in History & Philosophy of Science, C: Studies in History & Philosophy of Biological & Biomedical Sciences*, 35(2), 367–90.

Becker, Carol S. (1992), *Living and relating: An introduction to phenomenology* (Newbury Park, CA: SAGE).

Bell, Daniel (1973/1999), *The coming of post-industrial society: A venture in social forecasting* (New York: Basic).

Berner, Boel & Corinna Kruse (2013) (eds.), *Knowledge and evidence: Investigating technologies in practice* (Linköping: Department of Thematic Studies, Technology & Social Change, Linköping University).

Bohlin, Ingemar & Morten Sager (2011) (eds.), *Evidensens många ansikten: Evidensbaserad praktik i praktiken* (Lund: Arkiv).

Buckland, Michael K. (2012), 'What kind of science can information science be', *Journal of the American Society for Information Science & Technology*, 63(1), 1–7.

Carusi, Annamaria & Aud Sissel Hoel (2014), 'Toward a new ontology of scientific vision', in Catelijne Coopmans, Janet Vertesi, Michael E. Lynch & Steve Woolgar (eds.), *Representation in scientific practice revisited* (Cambridge: MIT Press).

Cole, Thomas R., Nathan S. Carlin & Ronald A. Carson (2015), *Medical humanities: An introduction* (Cambridge: CUP).

Drucker, Peter Ferdinand (1969), *The age of discontinuity: Guidelines to our changing society* (London: Pan).

Dumit, Joseph (2004), *Picturing personhood: Brain scans and diagnostic identity* (Princeton: PUP).

Eklöf, Motzi & Daniel Normark (2018), 'Den informatiska medicinen och ansvaret för den digitala patientens integritet', *Socialmedicinsk tidskrift*, 3, 345–55.

Engelbretsen, Eivind, Tony Joakim Sandset & John Ødemark (2017), 'Expanding the knowledge translation metaphor', *Health Research Policy & Systems*, 15(19).

Foucault, Michel (1980), *Power/knowledge: Selected interviews and other writings 1972–1977* (New York: Pantheon).

Frans, Emma (2017), *Larmrapporten* (Stockholm: Volante).

Frykman, Jonas & Nils Gilje (2003) (eds.), *Being there: New perspectives on phenomenology and the analysis of culture* (Lund: Nordic Academic Press).

Gottweis, Herbert (2008), 'Participation and the New Governance of Life', *BioSocieties*, 3(3), 265–86.

Gutting, Gary (2005), *Foucult: A very short introduction* (Oxford: OUP).

Hacking, Ian (1996), 'The looping effects of human kinds', in Dan Sperber, David Premack & Ann James Premack (eds.), *Causal cognition: A multidisciplinary debate* (Oxford: OUP).

Hansson, Kristofer & Karolina Lindh (2018), 'The hamburgers in the fridge: An interview with Professor Nikolas Rose about interdisciplinary collaboration, neuroscience and critical friendship', *Culture Unbound: Journal of Current Cultural Research*, 10(1), 115–22.

Hansson, Kristofer (2017), 'A different kind of engagement: P. C. Jersild's novel *A living soul*', in Kristofer Hansson & Markus Idvall (eds.), *Interpreting the brain in society: Cultural reflections on neuroscientific practices* (Lund: Arkiv förlag).

Hahn, Robert A. & Gaines, Atwood D. (eds.) (1985), Physicians of Western medicine: Anthropological approaches to theory and practice (Dordrecht: Reidel).

Haraway, Donna Jeanne (1985/2000), 'A cyborg manifesto: Science, technology, and socialist–feminism in the late twentieth century', *Posthumanism*, 69–84.

Husserl, Edmund (1972 [1913]), *Ideas: General introduction to pure phenomenology* (New York: Collier).

Ihde, Don (2012), *Experimental phenomenology: Multistabilities* (New York: State University of New York Press).

Jasanoff, Sheila (2004), *States of knowledge: The co-production of science and the social order* (London: Routledge).

Jordan, Brigitte (1983), *Birth in four cultures: [A crosscultural investigation of childbirth in Yucatan, Holland, Sweden and the United States]*. 3. ed. (Montréal: Eden P.).Keating,

Peter & Alberto Cambrosio (2006), *Biomedical platforms: Realigning the normal and the pathological in late twentieth-century medicine* (Cambridge, MA: MIT).

King, Alexandra Clare, Peter Orpin, Jessica Woodroffe & Kim Boyer (2017), 'Eating and ageing in rural Australia: Applying temporal perspectives from phenomenology to uncover meanings in older adults' experiences', *Ageing & Society*, 37(4), 753–76.

Kleinman, Arthur (1988), *The illness narratives: Suffering, healing, and the human condition* (New York: Basic).

Kristeva, Julia, Marie Rose Moro, John Ødemark & Eivind Engebretsen (2018), 'Cultural crossings of care: An appeal to the medical humanities', *Medical Humanities*, 44(1), 55–8.

Latour, Bruno (2003), 'Why has critique run out of steam? From matters of fact to matters of concern', *Critical Inquiry* [Special issue], 30(2), 25–248.

Latour, Bruno & Woolgar, Steve (1979), *Laboratory life: The social construction of scientific facts* (Beverly Hills: Sage).

Lyotard, Jean-François (1979), *La condition postmoderne: Rapport sur le savoir* (Paris: Éditions de Minuit).

Mishler, Elliot G. (ed.) (1981), *Social contexts of health, illness, and patient care* (Cambridge: Cambridge U. P.).

Mol, Annemarie (2008), *The logic of care: Health and the problem of patient choice* (Abingdon: Routledge).

Nichter, Mark & Lock , Margaret (eds.) (2002), *New horizons in medical anthropology: Essays in honour of Charles Leslie* (London: Routledge).

Nordgren, Lars & Kristofer Hansson (2019), 'Introductions' (eds.), *Health management: Vinst, värde, kvalitet i hälso- och sjukvård* (Stockholm: Sanoma utbildning).

Normark, Daniel (2019), 'Mobilising skill and making skill mobile: Crafoord's surgical tours in South America, 1950–1965', *Lychnos*, 127–149.

Östling, Johan, David Larsson Heidenblad & Anna Nilsson Hammar (2020) (eds.), *Forms of knowledge: Developing the history of knowledge* (Lund: Nordic Academic Press).

Pellizzoni, Luigi (2001), 'The myth of the best argument: Power, deliberation and reason', *British Journal of Sociology*, 52(1), 59–86.

Pickstone, John V. (2000), *Ways of knowing: A new history of science, technology and medicine* (Manchester: MUP).

Roberts, Albert R. & Yeager, Kenneth R. (eds.) (2006), *Foundations of evidence-based social work practice* (Oxford: Oxford University Press).

Rose, Nikolas (2007), *The politics of life itself: Biomedicine, power, and subjectivity in the twenty-first century* (Princeton: PUP).

Rose, Nikolas (2013), 'The human sciences in a biological age', *Theory, Culture & Society*, 30(1).

Rosenberg, William & Anna Donald (1995), 'Evidence based medicine: An approach to clinical problem-solving', *BMJ*, 310, 1122–6.

Schütz, Alfred & Talcott Parsons (1978), *The theory of social action: The correspondence of Alfred Schutz and Talcott Parsons* (Bloomington: Indiana University Press).

Secord, James A. (2004), 'Knowledge in transit', *Isis*, 94(4), 654–72.

Starr, Paul (1982), *The social transformation of American medicine* (New York: Basic Books).

Wiszmeg, Andréa (2017), 'Diffractions of the foetal cell suspension: Scientific knowledge and value in laboratory work', in Kristofer Hansson & Markus Idvall (eds.), *Interpreting the brain in society: Cultural reflections on neuroscientific practices* (Lund: Arkiv).

Wynne, Brian (1996), 'Misunderstood misunderstanding: Social identities and public uptake of science', in Alan Irwin & Brian Wynne (eds.), *Misunderstanding science? The public reconstruction of science and technology* (Cambridge: CUP).

PART I

MEDICAL KNOWLEDGE AND THE POLITICAL

CHAPTER 1

Prenatal diagnosis
The co-production of knowledge and values in medical research and public debate

Anna Tunlid

'Your money or your life—A consideration of prenatal diagnosis' ran the headline of an article published in several Swedish newspapers and magazines in the spring of 1978. It was written by three people with connections with the social care sector, and argued that prenatal diagnosis had profound social and moral consequences. It was now high time to have a wide-ranging debate about the values, justifications, and views underpinning its practice (Nordlund et al. 1978). The article was the prelude to an exhaustive public discussion about the direction, application and consequences of prenatal diagnosis. Developments in prenatal diagnosis had hitherto been a matter for the research community and the healthcare sector; now there was a demand for a broad public debate that could help shape national guidelines. This chapter shows how advanced medical technology such as prenatal diagnosis was discussed, evaluated, and renegotiated when translated from laboratories and clinics into the public arena and the debate about policy and regulation.[1]

The chapter draws on the theory of co-production, which describes how the development of scientific knowledge and its applications takes place in constant interactions with society's norms, values, and interests (Jasanoff 2004). Neither the production of knowledge nor its applications can be understood without considering the social and political contexts that are its preconditions. In this chapter, it is the movement of knowledge from research and clinical context out into public debate that is the main concern, and above all the question of policy. The focus is the notion of prenatal diagnostic practice represented by medical experts (medical researchers and doctors) and the views on prenatal diagnosis expressed in the media and in policy proposals. I analyse how notions of medical technology's practices and consequences were debated and questioned when medical knowledge moved from the laboratory and the clinic to the public sphere. When groups outside the research community debated prenatal diagnosis, other interpretive frameworks, contexts, and values were introduced, compared to those which had been central when the technology developed in the laboratories and the clinical context. The analysis shows there were different views about prenatal diagnosis in the public debate and the policy context, which differed somewhat from the medical experts' views. One conclusion of the present study is that the application and regulation of complex medical technologies require a continuous, unflinching public discussion in which both experts and representatives of different sections of civil society participate (Jasanoff 2005). Such discussions are the prerequisite for democratic decisions about biotechnologies which have the potential to influence people's fundamental ideas about *life itself* (Rose 2007), while at the same time retaining the scientific legitimacy of medicine.

The chapter covers a brief historical background and the broad outlines of the medical developments in prenatal diagnosis, before turning to the public debate and the official inquiry into prenatal diagnosis by the Swedish National Board of Health and Welfare in the early 1980s as part of the formulation of a national policy. First, the concept of co-production, and how it can be employed to understand what happens when knowledge moves between contexts, is discussed. The source material consists of articles in newspapers and magazines, particularly for the public debate, and the official inquiry proceedings, including the written responses by relevant organizations and government agencies; this material provides a broad cross-section of the opinions on prenatal diagnosis found in Swedish society in the late 1970s and early 1980s. Several opinions had historical resonances, expressing historically-shaped notions of health and disease, deviation and normality. The historical perspective can therefore help conceptualize how medical knowledge has evolved, stabilized and changed, not only in its translation from one context to the next, but also between different periods.

The embeddedness of knowledge

There is a well-established notion in the history of science and science and technology studies that knowledge is embedded—that its content cannot be separated from the social, political, and cultural contexts in which it is produced and applied. The context plays a role, both for the knowledge produced and for how that knowledge is perceived, applied, and used. One expression of this is Sheila Jasanoff's concept of co-production:

> the ways in which we know and represent the world (both nature and society) are inseparable from the ways in which we choose to live in it. Knowledge and its material embodiments are at once products of social work and constitutive of forms of social life; society cannot function without knowledge any more than knowledge can exist without appropriate social support. Scientific knowledge, in particular, is not a transcendent mirror of reality. It both embeds and is embedded in social practices, identities, norms, conventions, discourses, instruments and institutions—in short, in all building blocks of what we term the *social*. (Jasanoff 2004, 2–3)

Our knowledge and our ideas about the world cannot be disconnected from the society in which we live. Biomedical knowledge produced in a laboratory or any other research environment is equally part of its social, meaning-making context. This means that when this knowledge is translated from knowledge-producing to applied knowledge contexts, it will both influence and be influenced by the latter context. Co-production is therefore a useful perspective for understanding how social, political, and cultural values interact with knowledge in the phases of its construction, mobilization, and application, wherever in society it is (see Lindh in this volume).

According to Jasanoff, some situations lend themselves to making the embedded nature of knowledge visible. One is when new technologies are established, questioned, stabilized, and eventually regulated in a society. Prenatal diagnosis was just such a technology. It was developed in a scientific and medical context moulded by certain views and values; when it became the subject of public debate, it came up against differing views and values. This was particularly true of views on people with disabilities, but also opinions on what constitutes human life, reproductive rights, and the direction of future medical research. The debate about prenatal diagnosis thus not only shows how new technology is discussed and questioned when it moves out of the laboratory or clinic, it also shows that when a new, complex technology is introduced, a variety of social, political, and ethical views are mobilized, which will be discussed in this chapter.

The historical roots of prenatal diagnosis

Prenatal diagnosis developed from knowledge in such disciplines as medical genetics, clinical chemistry, and obstetrics, of which the advances in medical genetics played a significant role, as the diagnosis of genetic diseases was a major part of the first prenatal diagnoses. One particularly important discovery was made in 1956, when the geneticists Albert Levan and Joe Hin Tjio found that humans have 46 chromosomes, not 48 as thought (Harper 2006). Three years later, the French paediatrician and geneticist Jérôme Lejeune and his co-workers suggested that Down's syndrome was caused by an extra chromosome. The same year, 1959, it was found that Turner's syndrome and Klinefelter's syndrome are both sex chromosome disorders, and the following year further links were found between chromosomal abnormalities and specific syndromes (Kevles 1995; Lindee 2005; Löwy 2017).

At first this new genetic knowledge was used to diagnose patients or confirm diagnoses, and soon it came into use in genetic counselling, which became established at a handful of hospitals in Sweden (Björkman & Tunlid 2017). The background of genetic counselling can be found not only in the emerging field of medical genetics, but also in the eugenics movement of the early twentieth century, with the latter's aim of controlling the genetic composition of the population (Broberg & Tydén 2005).[2] An important element in Swedish eugenics was the 1934 and 1941 Sterilization Acts, which allowed for sterilization of individuals classified as legally incompetent without their consent.[3] A group that was specifically targeted was the 'feeble-minded', who were judged to be genetically inferior and a social and economic burden on society, and whose procreation was assumed to weaken the population's genetic composition (Tydén 2002). Eugenics, however, was a multifaceted movement that was not only government-driven; the spread of eugenic ideas in Swedish society meant that individuals learnt of the significance of their genetic inheritance, and turned to genetic experts for advice on reproductive health (Björkman 2015). Often they were afraid they might have children with disabilities or serious diseases.

In developing medical genetics and genetic counselling in the post-war period, many geneticists emphasized the individual's right to make their own decisions and asserted that counselling was not intended to improve the heredity of the population. Most historians agree, however, that eugenic ideas and practices did not end with the Second World War (Bashford 2010). Exactly which parts of the eugenic mindset were abandoned and which were transformed and lived on into our own time with its ever more advanced genetic and reproductive technologies is much debated. As the historian of biology Nathaniel Comfort (2012) suggests, perhaps 'the eugenic impulse'—the urge to eliminate disease, improve health, and reduce suffering by controlling human heredity—has been one of the most enduring in this history. It certainly comes with a variety of sociocultural values about what constitutes good health, well-being, and quality of life, married with the wish to choose certain traits and reject abnormalities and diseases when making reproductive decisions. As will be seen, it was around these choices that much of the debate about prenatal diagnosis revolved.

From statistical risks to information about the foetus

Before the advent of prenatal diagnosis in the 1970s, the methods available to geneticists for genetic counselling were based on statistical analyses of the risk that parents would pass on a certain disease or disability to their children. These estimates were based on known inheritance mechanisms and experience-based knowledge of how diseases were inherited. Armed with this knowledge and a map of the family's disease patterns, the geneticist calculated the risk of a hereditary disease being passed to any future children. Those who received genetic counselling were thus told there was a risk, expressed as a percentage, of passing a specific disease or disability to their children. This figure for risk was what parents had to consider when contemplating pregnancy.

The point of genetic counselling, according to the Swedish paediatrician and medical geneticist Karl-Henrik Gustavson, was 'to provide factual information about the hereditary or non-hereditary nature of the disease and to communicate how great the risk will be for subsequent children' (Gustavson 1967). According to Gustavson, genetic counselling had no eugenic purpose, and existed only to help individuals or families with their 'special problems'. The notion that patient autonomy would be respected was often emphasized to underline it was the interests of the woman and the family which were paramount, not the state. The genetic counsellor's job was to provide the woman with objective, neutral information, and not to influence her position on a new pregnancy. However, Gustavson and other genetic counsellors knew the risk figures on which they based their advice could be difficult for laypeople to grasp, as there were such variations in people's notions of significant and minor risk or the severity of a disease or birth defect. Moreover, parents often felt guilt and shame about the risk of passing on hereditary diseases or disabilities to their children (Gustavson 1967; Lindsten et al. 1975). In practice, genetic counselling was a very complex business, open to interpretation and value judgements. Risk calculations could be presented in different ways, as could information about the diseases or disabilities concerned. Medical knowledge thus came to be embedded in certain notions of disease, abnormality, and normality that were largely characterized by medical expertise.

The circumstances in which women made reproductive decisions changed dramatically in the early 1970s with prenatal diagnosis, made possible by medical genetics and the invention or improvement of several medical technologies. One of these was amniocentesis, a procedure in which a small amount of the amniotic fluid is removed from the amniotic sac. In the late 1950s it was found that the cells in the amniotic fluid could be used for foetal sex determination—knowledge that was central to the diagnosis of sex-linked hereditary diseases. However, it was only in the late 1960s that cells were first cultured from the amniotic fluid, which was crucial for analysing chromosomes. Another important technology in this context was medical ultrasound, which in the early 1970s improved the ability to withdraw amniotic fluid (Löwy 2017).

If a woman underwent prenatal diagnosis, the information she was given no longer concerned the risk of a particular disease, but the specific condition of the foetus she was carrying. Amniocentesis made it possible to detect chromosomal abnormalities and determine the foetal sex. Doctors were also able to diagnose a number of unusual but serious metabolic disorders and to establish if there was a risk of spina bifida, a neural tube defect. Instead of multiple or complex risk figures, a woman who underwent prenatal diagnosis and found that the foetus had a disease or condition could decide whether to terminate the pregnancy.

The development of prenatal diagnosis occurred in parallel with calls for more liberal abortion laws in Sweden (Lennerhed 2017). Under the 1938 Abortion Act, there was the possibility of legal abortion, but only in certain circumstances: the woman had to apply for an abortion, and it could be granted only with reference to certain specific indications.[4] One was the 'eugenic indication', which meant the risk that a parent would transmit 'insanity, mental retardation, or severe physical disease'. In 1963, in the wake of the thalidomide tragedy, foetal defects were added as an indication. Although the number of abortions on eugenic grounds declined in the post-war period (Tydén 2002), abortion due to a suspected hereditary disease or condition was a well-established practice in the Swedish health service.

In 1974, a new Abortion Act was passed that gave the woman the right to elect to have an abortion up to 18 weeks of pregnancy, after which an abortion was only permitted in exceptional circumstances with the permission of the National Board of Health and Welfare.[5] Permission could be given until the foetus was considered viable, which in practice meant the end of 22 weeks. The majority of applications for abortion due to a birth defect were granted by the National Board of Health and Welfare, since the test results of the prenatal diagnosis were usually not available until after 18 weeks of pregnancy. Abortions due to diagnosed foetal defects were called selective abortions, distinguishing them from the general abortions when the pregnancy was unwanted.

The introduction of prenatal diagnosis

Prenatal diagnosis was introduced in the Swedish health service in the early 1970s. It was primarily offered to pregnant women over a certain age (it had long been known that the risk of Down's syndrome increased with maternal age) and women with disability or genetic disease in the family. A third group was women who, for other reasons, had strong concerns about having a child with a disability or genetic disease.

Prenatal diagnosis was thus targeted at individuals and families in specific situations. It was seen by doctors as helping women in the designated risk groups by detecting several serious hereditary diseases and disabilities early in pregnancy, and meant that a foetus with one of those diseases or a chromosome abnormality could be aborted if the woman so wished, while an abortion could be avoided if the foetus was healthy. Families who ran a high risk of having a child with a disability or genetic disease could thus be 'guaranteed that any future child would not have the hereditary disease for which they had an increased risk' according to some of the leading doctors in the field (Kjessler et al. 1972, 2362): their view was that prenatal diagnosis led to greater numbers of healthy children being born, and a reduction in the number of abortions of healthy foetuses. The new technology was thus described by the doctors as improving women's opportunities to make informed reproductive choices. However, it could also be described as the prospect of greatly reducing 'the number of hereditarily defective children' (*Svenska Dagbladet* 17 Mar. 1971). In a letter to the National Board of Health, three doctors argued that prenatal diagnosis should be extended as follows:

> Through prenatal diagnosis, parents can be reassured early in pregnancy with accurate information. If the expected child is healthy, one can thus avoid the abortion of a healthy foetus. If the diagnosis of the child is positive, and if the mother wishes to terminate the pregnancy, society can be expected to save significant sums, which would otherwise be needed for the future institutional care of the defective child. If only a small proportion of the money so saved is made available for prenatal diagnosis, something of benefit to both individual and society could be achieved satisfactorily.[6]

The reproductive choices of women and families were expected to fall into line with society's interest in cutting the costs of healthcare and social care for disabled and seriously ill children. The expense of expanding prenatal diagnosis and genetic counselling could therefore be justified on socio-economic grounds, compared with the costs of health and social care (Lindsten et al. 1976).

The possibility of using prenatal diagnosis to prevent the birth of children with disabilities was noted in several contexts. In Sweden's medical journal, *Läkartidningen*, two paediatricians, Bengt Hagberg and Karl-Henrik Gustavson, expressed the hope that prenatal diagnosis would progress to the point where a simple blood test early in pregnancy would detect if the foetus had Down's syndrome. It was their belief that 'a preventive approach' to mental disability was justified not only on humanitarian grounds but also on financial ones. According to their calculations, the cost to the taxpayer of a single 'severely mentally disturbed child' in institutional care was SEK 1.2 million a decade (Hagberg & Gustavson 1978). It is unclear what they meant by humanitarian grounds, but it may have been both the family's situation and the child's, as doctors often said that disabilities and hereditary diseases caused suffering to both children and families.

The early discourse of prenatal diagnosis, in which doctors and medical experts took the lead, therefore had several elements. It was based on medical advances which gave women greater opportunities to make reproductive choices, but it also plainly involved value judgements about serious diseases and disabilities. The individual's right to choose in the question of abortion was combined with a belief that there was a public interest in reducing the number of people with genetic diseases or disabilities. The discourse also spanned such notions as disease, suffering, and normality. Children with genetic diseases and disabilities were often described as defective, and their condition a source of suffering for them and their families. Prenatal diagnosis, combined with abortion, was seen as a way of preventing this suffering. In this way the new technology was placed in a context characterized by certain norms and values.

When medical notions of foetal diagnosis were debated more generally, it was primarily in terms of two contemporary discourses: one that stressed women's rights to make independent, well-informed choices about reproductive issues, and one about perceptions of people with disabilities and their place in society. Alongside this was a discourse about the right to abortion per se, but it hardly featured in the debate under consideration here. There was no organized anti-abortion movement in Sweden at this time, although there was a belief, especially in Christian contexts, that abortion rights should be restricted.[7]

Public interest in prenatal diagnosis

At first, the debate about prenatal diagnosis was limited to the medical context, with a few exceptions (see Gustafson 1980). An early attempt to address the wider implications of the technology was mounted by the Liberal politician Kerstin Anér in a high-profile motion in Parliament in 1972 on the inviolability of the individual, in which she stressed that society faced a difficult, complex situation because of recent medical and technological advances. One was prenatal diagnosis, which according to Anér could soon lead to the question of whether it was a right for all pregnant women to be informed of any genetic diseases, and whether that right would bring with it a duty to abort any foetus with a defect. Anér asked whether 'society would be the child's advocate and say you have the right to live; or you have the right not to live'. The motion resulted in a proposal to set up a working group to discuss the social and legal consequences of medical developments, and whether there were grounds to impose any restrictions on medical research (Anér 1972). After an extensive consultation process, the parliamentary motion was rejected.[8]

There had been little public discussion, though, by the time 'Your money or your life' was published in the spring of 1978. The debate which the article sparked, and the demand for practice guidelines for prenatal diagnosis from the medical authorities, led the National Board of Health and Welfare to appoint an official inquiry in 1980. It brought together doctors and other medical experts to clarify and describe the central issues of prenatal diag-nosis. As the Director General of the National Board of Health and

Welfare said, the advances in medical research had determined the direction taken, and now it was important to clarify whether society should influence future developments (Socialstyrelsen 1982). The inquiry's interim report addressed both the medical and technical aspects of prenatal diagnosis and the psychological, ethical, and legal ramifications. It also asked several questions about the application of prenatal diagnosis. The interim report was circulated for public consultation to various public authorities and organizations as normal, resulting in the submission of a very large number of official consultation responses.

The public debate, like the consultation responses, addressed a range of broader issues and problematics. In what follows, three central themes in this material have been singled out. First, the importance of prenatal diagnosis for views on people with disabilities and the socio-economics. Second, foetal rights and the situations in which it was right to terminate a pregnancy—a theme that tied in with the public debate about abortion per se, and also the question of prenatal diagnosis and selective abortion. Third, the implementation and regulation of prenatal diagnosis, including whether there were reasons to change the standing abortion legislation, a theme with a bearing on reproductive rights as formulated in the 1974 Abortion Act. Also considered here is the side theme of the nature of medical research, and whether there was reason to redirect or limit the research relating to prenatal diagnosis.

Prenatal diagnosis and disability

The article 'Your Money or Your Life' dealt pointedly with the three points that the authors said had been the key arguments for prenatal diagnosis: reducing the suffering of families with children with disabilities, reducing the suffering of the child, and reducing the cost to society. To the first argument, the authors said that the remedies were social measures and changed attitudes. The idea that prenatal diagnosis could reduce the suffering of people with disabilities was also called into question, because only those with a disability or their immediate relatives could decide what constituted a meaningful life. However, according to the authors, the humanitarian arguments were overshadowed by the third argument concerning economics, and they cautioned that in a society driven by profitability, efficiency, and the rational use of resources, people with disabilities were dismissed as unprofitable. According to them, this was the chief reason for offering prenatal diagnosis (Nordlund et al. 1978).

The claim that the impetus behind prenatal diagnosis was socio-economic outraged several doctors, who countered that the primary reason was to reduce the suffering of children with severe congenital diseases, disabilities, or birth defects, and the same went for families too. It should be noted here that suffering would be alleviated by the abortion of foetuses with those diagnoses—there was no possibility of treatment in utero. Furthermore, according to the doctors, the possibility of prenatal diagnosis would allay the fears of parents worried about future pregnancies. The socio-economic arguments were now toned down and the medical and humanitarian aims emphasized (Gustavson 1978; Kjessler 1979). However, even among doctors there were those who wondered whether Down's syndrome could justify abortion on the basis of diminished suffering. Stig Melander, a senior consultant at the department of obstetrics and gynaecology in Norrköping, wrote that 'It is a widely accepted fact that the mongoloid as a conscious, living person does not suffer to any appreciable extent from his condition' (Melander 1978). Despite this, an increasing number of pregnancies were terminated due to Down's syndrome, and it could not be ruled out that this affected people with disabilities:

> The hardest thing for many people, as for me, however, is the idea of those disabled individuals who have already been born, who are aware of their situation. How can the disabled view this state of affairs, this reasoning, as anything other than deeply humiliating and offensive? If I were on the way now, would you others have made sure I never came into the world? I am a deeply unwelcome

citizen. Can anyone help convince me that I don't look at them this way? (Melander 1978)

The Swedish disability movement was divided in their view of prenatal diagnosis. The reasons for and against were many, and related to attitudes towards people with disabilities and the support for them and their families. Many parents of children with disabilities found there were major deficiencies in social support, and the pressure on them to take care of their disabled children themselves was at times described as 'an unreasonable workload' (*Dagens Nyheter* 10 June 1980). From this perspective, the possibility of prenatal diagnosis could be felt important for future pregnancies. Yet there was a strong concern within the movement that prenatal diagnosis would end in quality checks on all foetuses, with people with disabilities thought an undesirable group in society. Another concern was that the voluntary nature of testing and abortion would be eroded: prenatal diagnosis might seem obligatory rather than an option, and abortion the self-evident choice if a disease or disability were diagnosed.

At first, however, the disability movement was cautiously positive about prenatal diagnosis. In the early 1970s, the Swedish National Association for People with Intellectual Disability (FUB), which largely organized parents who had children with disabilities, argued that genetic counselling should be expanded, because many of its members were worried about having another child with the same diagnosis. Over the 1970s, though, fears grew that prenatal diagnosis would lead to selection and eventually the emergence of an elite society. In essence, the disability movement tried to defend the rights of people with disabilities while supporting access to prenatal diagnosis for individual families. Prenatal diagnosis could be justified on an individual basis, whenever the expectant parents felt themselves incapable of caring for a child with a disability. 'We couldn't cope having another mongoloid child', as one parent put it (Wahlström 1974). The debate within the FUB became more heated in the late 1970s when the question of human dignity and societal issues was raised. Prenatal diagnosis was said to be 'not primarily a question for experts—but about views on human dignity and what kind of society we really want' (*FUB-kontakt* 1978). FUB representatives rejected the standard argument that prenatal diagnosis could prevent suffering. For example, it was indefensible to say that all children with Down's syndrome suffered, and it was virtually impossible to know in advance what life would be like for them (*Stockholms-Tidningen* 22 Nov. 1982).

In its official consultation response to the National Board of Health and Welfare's report, the FUB stated that it represented an uncompromising view of humankind: 'Each person has a unique value in themselves. Even a severely disabled person has an infinite value, and the right to our respect and love.'[9] Any tendency to question the right to be born or to live with full human rights, regardless of disability, had to be fought, and efforts had to continue to direct research and find resources to provide life chances for children with disabilities and their families. However, the possibility of prenatal diagnosis could not be rejected. According to the FUB, Sweden's abortion legislation and the rules on free abortion were incompatible with the prohibition on abortion on the basis of birth defects; it stressed, however, that its position had nothing to do with the attributes of the foetus, but on the family's situation, and whether the woman judged that the family had the resources for a child who required extra care.

Likewise, the Swedish Disability Federation Central Committee (HCK), an umbrella body for several disability organizations, was initially in favour of prenatal diagnosis, arguing it could prevent disability (Gustafson 1980, 66). However, by the time of its official consultation response to the National Board of Health and Welfare's report, the HCK, much like the FUB, emphasized the equal right to dignity and that society had to provide support so everyone would have equal treatment.[10] The HCK could not accept prenatal diagnosis 'designed to sift out the people who will not be allowed to live'. Nor should the severity of the birth defect determine whether an abortion was defensible. For the HCK, the ethical issue was not one of degree; the conflict existed in the idea that one could 'quality 'assess' a foetus. Rather, it emphasized the importance of changing society so the consequences of disabilities could be compensated for or prevented. Many of the HCK's members were worried that tolerance of people with disabilities would wane and that society's resources for the group would stagnate or be cut. That said, it did not reject prenatal diagnosis out of hand. What it objected to was prenatal diagnosis predicated on the abortion of all foetuses with a defect. However, it could support 'foetal-focused therapy', or prenatal diagnosis focused on the treatment of foetuses.

Segments of the disability movement clearly distanced themselves from prenatal diagnosis, however. For example, the Swedish Association of the Visually Impaired 'forcefully' rejected

> all prenatal diagnosis designed to cull human populations. No disability could possibly justify abortion in a democratic society. Any other approach can have devastating effects on how people with disabilities are viewed. But it can also lead to the foundations of democracy and views on people and people's worth are changing beyond recognition.[11]

There may have been several reasons for the disability movement's varied views on prenatal diagnosis. One was that the associations of parents of children with disabilities were often more cautiously positive than those associations of people with disabilities (Gustafson 1984). Being the parent of a disabled person often carried great responsibility. Attitudes may also have been affected by the severity of the disability. Although several associations objected to rating various disabilities and conditions, that did not rule out that parents who already had children with very severe disabilities and significant care needs were in favour of prenatal diagnosis.

The socio-economic arguments, though, were firmly and unanimously rejected by the disability movement. In the early 1980s that case was still being made, with talk of cost–benefit analyses and calculations of the economic gains to be had from the increased diagnosis of birth defects and subsequent abortions and saved care costs. 'However you want to count it, prenatal diagnosis is very profitable for society', as a county council politician put it (Åkerman 1982; *FUB-kontakt* 1982). Disgust at this sort of calculation went far beyond the disability movement: it opened for 'general hatred of disabilities', wrote the Social Democratic newspaper *Stockholms-Tidningen* (5 July 1982), which thought the question ought to be discussed in terms of society's general support for people with disabilities. Only societies which included them could avoid prenatal diagnosis becoming an instrument for selecting and removing 'non-perfect' people.

Foetal rights

Another theme in the debate about prenatal diagnosis was the rights of the foetus and the ability to diagnose and possibly treat foetuses with birth defects. As the conservative newspaper *Svenska Dagbladet* (9 Dec. 1979) said, this could reasonably be expected to raise the ethical question of whether the foetus is a person with the right to life and not part of the woman's body. The Swedish Medical Society reasoned along similar lines in its views on the ethics of prenatal diagnosis, stating that the possibility not only of diagnosing but also treating foetuses would probably lead to the rights of the foetus as an independent individual being respected to a greater extent 'than is now the case' (Svenska Läkaresällskapets delegation för medicinsk etik 1980). Before the new Abortion Act was passed in 1974, the Medical Society's Delegation for Medical Ethics had stated that the foetus had its own life, and that as a potential human should be given legal protection; however, it was omitted from the new legislation (Svenska Läkaresällskapets delegation för medicinsk etik 1979). Thus, it was a view that enjoyed a resurgence because of the ability to diagnose and possibly treat in utero. The debate about prenatal diagnosis therefore evolved to include the question of when the human embryo could be regarded as having personhood.

This and many other issues were covered by a special inquiry on the medical ethical aspects of prenatal diagnosis appointed by the Swedish national synod in 1979.[12] Medical experts as well as theologians sat on the inquiry panel.[13] As described in their report, prenatal diagnosis had three aims: to prevent the abortion of healthy foetuses; to develop methods for treating foetuses before any permanent damage; and to provide a basis for a decision to possibly terminate a pregnancy. These were the three aims doctors had always recognized. The synod inquiry was unanimous that the first two aims could be accepted without reservation, so it concentrated on the third—abortions after prenatal diagnosis. Opinion was divided on these so-called selective abortions, but the synod inquiry could agree that they were part of 'the much larger and ultimately fundamental problem of abortion' (Fagerberg 1980, 8). It amounted to the foetus's right to life. Prenatal diagnosis was thus tied to the questions of the point at which the fertilized egg or embryo had personhood and at what point it merited protection. This went hand in hand with an ongoing debate about euthanasia—the circumstances in which it was right to actively end a life—and the 1974 Abortion Act, which, according to the synod inquiry, had not addressed the rights of the foetus. The synod inquiry's various positions on these questions were summarized by the chairman of the Swedish Medical Society's Delegation for Medical Ethics, who hoped that a 'more thorough and nuanced discussion of abortion than the one which preceded the 1974 decision would now be possible' (Giertz 1980, 117).

However, according to the synod inquiry, selective abortions were, to some extent, special compared to general abortions. The pregnancy was initially desired, but the foetus was found to have a disease or defect. Further, they were often performed late in pregnancy. 'In these circumstances, no one can ignore the fact that life is extinguished because it is not desirable', said Gustav Giertz, physician and chairman of the Swedish Medical Society's Delegation for Medical Ethics (Giertz 1980, 119). The synod inquiry could not agree on whether such abortions should be considered ethically defensible or not. Views ranged from certainty that the Abortion Act accurately reflected current norms to calls to safeguard the rights of the foetus and a belief that abortion was only ethically acceptable

46

under special conditions such as incurable and fatal birth defects or danger to the mother's physical or mental health. The synod inquiry did not believe the Abortion Act should be changed, but did not preclude a situation when diseases of the foetus could not only be diagnosed but also treated, meaning that the legal status of the foetus as an independent individual would have to command far greater respect. According to Archbishop Olof Sundby, advances in prenatal diagnosis had reinforced an awareness of the respect for the life of the foetus (*Upsala Nya Tidning* 17 June 1980). The inquiry attracted considerable attention, placed the foetal rights on the agenda, and by extension fuelled the wider debate about prenatal diagnosis and abortion (*Dagens Nyheter* 17 June 1980; *Svenska Dagbladet* 18 June 1980). The medical knowledge generated by prenatal diagnosis as it moved to other contexts than its original genetic, medical context thus prompted new questions—or brought to life old ones—of which several concerned conflicting norms and values.

Practice and regulation

When prenatal diagnosis was introduced in the Swedish health service, it was with no specific guidelines or regulations. Much of the public debate had turned on the question of how prenatal diagnosis would be implemented, what would be allowed, and whether specific regulations were required besides the 1974 Abortion Act. Many of the voices in the debate were worried about what the future held. The liberal newspaper *Dagens Nyheter* wondered whether prenatal diagnosis could become mandatory, and what choices parents would be faced with: 'Will the authorities permit diagnosed harmful genes to be reproduced? Will the taxpayer, who will foot the bill, tolerate that foetuses suspected to be defective become people?' (*Dagens Nyheter* 18 June 1980). The eugenicist mindset was cited as a warning lesson. The disability movement also demanded regulation. According to the HCK's registrar, Rolf Utberg, not every disease was grounds for abortion. As he wrote, 'I believe that all kinds of people should be welcome and that we should have very strict rules for how prenatal diagnosis should be conducted' (*Dagens Nyheter* 27 July 1982).

The question of guidelines or regulations was also raised by the National Board of Health and Welfare in its inquiry into prenatal diagnosis. Who should be offered prenatal diagnosis? Was there cause to change the 1974 Abortion Act? Should a woman have the right to choose, even if the reason for an abortion was the foetus's attributes? On the first question, many consultation bodies—except those which flatly rejected prenatal diagnosis—accepted the practice developed by the Swedish health service of prenatal diagnosis being offered to special risk groups. However, segments of the disability movement were critical of the concept of 'risk groups', which often featured in the debate, and argued vigilance was needed so attitudes towards people with disabilities would not gradually worsen.[14] In medical quarters, meanwhile, the view was that fear and anxiety felt by women was as important a reason for prenatal diagnosis, and that any rules had to be adaptable to the individual situation.[15] It is interesting to note that in its consultation response to the National Board of Health and Welfare's report, the Swedish Medical Association argued that the final rules for prenatal diagnosis and the resources it would attract should be the subject of a broad parliamentary inquiry, as 'the correct democratic approach'.[16] This was not detailed in the consultation response opinion, but was in line with views expressed by individual doctors (*Dagens Nyheter* 23 July 1982), perhaps an indication of the need for clinical praxis consistent with society's values and norms.

Thus while the majority of consultation bodies believed that prenatal diagnosis should be available to certain groups, many were critical of screening, with all pregnant women offered the tests to detect serious birth defects.[17] Several consultation bodies stressed that prenatal diagnosis had to be voluntary, and if it came to screening it could impose such pressure on women that in practice it would be difficult to say no. Even voluntary testing made some uneasy, not least in the disability movement, for whom just the offer of prenatal diagnosis was problematic, concerned that in practice women did not have freedom of choice. It could be difficult to refuse. 'The entirety of the technological situation with its (ostensible) accuracy and effectiveness exerts a strong manipulative influence. There is little scope for questioning, reflection, and emotional evaluation. It is simplest and best to let technology have its way', wrote the Swedish Heart and Lung Association.[18] According to the National Association of the Disabled, if a foetus was found to have defects abortion was not voluntary, as there was a very strong pressure on the woman in this situation to abort, something that the National Board of Health and Welfare (Socialstyrelsen 1982, 81) also noted in its report.[19]

The question of altering the right to free abortion was closely linked to rapid medical developments, which meant that an increasing number of foetal diseases and abnormalities could be diagnosed ever earlier. According to the inquiry, there was an evident risk of 'quality checks' on the foetus and a greater number of abortions for less serious abnormalities. The measures considered included the possibility of increased surveillance of abortions due to birth defects, and partial restrictions on the right to have an abortion due to birth defects. Regarding surveillance of abortions due to birth defects, the inquiry asked whether a woman who wanted to have an abortion between weeks 14 and 18 of pregnancy should have to state her reason. Since the results of prenatal diagnosis were rarely available before the end of week 18, the majority of abortions due to birth defects were decided by the National Board of Health and Welfare (though in principle it always gave permission); they therefore had a good overview of the reasons given. If more birth defects were diagnosed before week 18, the inquiry feared this supervisory aspect would be lost 'unless special steps were taken'. At least initially, the proposal that a reason would have to be given for an abortion between weeks 14 and 18 was not designed to limit a woman's right to an abortion. However, future changes were not ruled out (Socialstyrelsen 1982, 106).

By extension, the inquiry foresaw 'bigger problems' arising from future medical developments, namely that minor abnormalities would increasingly be detectable. Would this justify imposing limits, deciding which birth defects would be considered valid grounds for an abortion? The inquiry emphasized that regulation would scarcely be possible without overruling women's autonomy, and it therefore asked whether abortion on the grounds of birth defects was such a problem it justified tearing up the basic principle of the abortion legislation, namely a woman's right to choose. Was it the woman's right alone to decide to have an abortion, even when the reason was the foetus's traits?

To check the reasons for abortions between weeks 14 and 18 or to restrict the woman's right to choose would require changes to free access to abortion. Most consultation bodies strongly opposed any such restrictions, and especially the majority of the women's movement, the campaign for the 1974 Abortion Act fresh in their minds. This did not prevent many women's organizations commenting on the National Board of Health and Welfare's report that it was an ethically complex issue, which would affect society's views on disability.[20] Social Democratic Women in Sweden was one organization to emphasize that for decades women had fought for the right to abortion, including the right to decide without giving a reason. They did not agree that the fundamentals of the 1974 Abortion Act had changed.

> *Then as now*, we hold that in balancing the foetus's right to development on the one hand and its right to be born into human dignity, the latter must weigh more heavily. *Then as now*, we contend it is the mother alone who can determine whether the conditions of human dignity can be met.[21]

Even the Fredrika Bremer Association, one of the oldest Swedish women's organizations, stressed the importance of free abortion: 'Now, as before, we wish to state our belief that a woman's right to decide about the possible termination of a pregnancy may not be limited.' For them it was 'obvious that the woman bases her judgement about a possible termination of a pregnancy on whether she can, whether she dares, assume responsibility for the child … Who better than the woman to judge what she can cope with.'[22] The Women's Political Committee of the Left Party Communists also stressed women's ability 'if supported to take difficult decisions', and there was no reason whatsoever to restrict the 1974 Abortion Act in the light of advances in prenatal diagnosis. It could not be construed any other way 'than as a distrust of a woman's ability to decide for herself on what conditions she wants to give birth.'[23] The women's political association that most disapproved of prenatal diagnosis was, not surprisingly, the Christian Democratic Women's Association, their view being coloured by their general dislike of the 1974 Abortion Act. Their precept was the sanctity of life and the equal dignity of all, and they believed abortion was a last resort.[24]

One of the most determined defenders of a woman's right to choose was the Swedish Association for Sexuality Education (RFSU), a non-profit organization that had long championed the right to free abortion. For the RFSU it was unthinkable that a woman should have to request an abortion because of minor abnormalities other than in purely exceptional cases, and to change the regulations for abortions in weeks 14 to 18, as the inquiry discussed, would be to reimpose on the woman 'a paternalism that after a long struggle she had finally rid herself of with the 1974 Abortion Act'. The very idea 'that once again she would be declared not to be trusted to decide a thing that so deeply impinges on her life' was offensive in the extreme. Worse, if it were possible to ban abortions for minor birth defects, the RFSU feared that it could end in a ban on all abortions where there was no birth defect. In other words, it was a direct threat to the right to free abortion.[25]

The doctors too defended the existing abortion legislation and a woman's right to choose, even when the reason was the foetus's condition. This was in line with current rules, and 'all our other legislation in the field of healthcare is predicated on it being the adult who has to take decisions.'[26]

With few exceptions, the right to free abortion thus went unchallenged by the debate about prenatal diagnosis. But many expressed restrictive views about access to prenatal diagnosis, and called for vigilance about the technology's ethical and social consequences, and the importance of greater support for people with disabilities and their families.

Freedom of research and its consequences

Throughout the debate on prenatal diagnosis, new research findings and methods were published. This, combined with medical experts' hopes that in the future even more diseases and conditions could be diagnosed and that some treatment in utero would be possible, meant that terms such as foetal medicine, foetal therapy, and foetal surgery were introduced into the debate, largely to argue that prenatal diagnosis was not merely a question of birth defects and abortion. Existing fears persisted that such developments might have undesirable effects, especially in negative views of disability and the pursuit of 'perfect children'. The issue of research funding and whether it should be regulated was therefore part of the debate about prenatal diagnosis. The National Board of Health and Welfare's report acknowledged that independent research would lead in directions which, for a variety of reasons could have no application in society, and asked whether the applications or the research itself should be controlled in any way (Socialstyrelsen 1982, ii–iii). This part of the debate reflected an awareness that knowledge production in prenatal diagnosis was associated with strongly held values and norms.

Medical experts and researchers, naturally enough, opposed controls on research: the positive effects of prenatal diagnosis outweighed even the ethical problems posed by new knowledge and techniques.[27] Any attempt to control independent research would be unfortunate. Instead, what was needed was preparedness to manage the social and ethical problems that arose.[28] The disability movement, meanwhile, had a more restrictive stance. It was widely felt that resources should be channelled to research on the prevention and treatment of birth defects—to foetal therapy, in other words. Many also pointed to the importance of research and measures that made it possible for people with disabilities to live in the community. Few opposed the idea that research should be independent, but many were critical of the lack of reflection and democratic discussion about its practical implications. This was the view of the Swedish Association of the Visually Impaired, among others: 'We find it horrifying that such important research as lies behind prenatal diagnosis can be developed and put to practical use before society's decision-making organs even have the chance to evaluate it and decide.'[29] Medical knowledge production should not be allowed without in-depth, democratic discussions about the possible consequences when that knowledge is transferred from the laboratory to the clinical setting. As these comments demonstrate, what was asked for was a democratic conversation, a form of public engagement with science (Irwin et al. 2013; see also Lindh in this volume), where knowledge was not only translated between different contexts, but also subjected to discussion, criticism, and reflection.

Conclusions

This chapter examines the new interpretations and understandings of prenatal diagnosis when it was translated from the medical and clinical context to the public sphere. The public debate was influenced by several movements of the day—the disability movement, the women's movement—and also by enduring historical trends in views on health and disease, normality and deviation. The early medical discourse, which acknowledged the opportunities to reject foetuses diagnosed with genetic diseases and chromosomal abnormalities, thus reducing suffering and increasing the proportion of healthy children, was challenged by the debate about human dignity and everyone's right to live an equal and dignified life. Soon the complexities accelerated as the debate opened up to include everything from ethical issues to political problems, and ultimately whether there were reasons to limit prenatal diagnosis in practice and to impose restrictions on the existing abortion legislation, which, after long investigations and discussions, had been passed just a decade before.

That there were deep reservations about a new, far-reaching technology during its introduction was not in itself strange. According to Jasanoff (2004), this stage, when the social order of technology has not yet stabilized, is when it is usual for conflicts over its interpretation, values, and standardization. Questions, debate, should be thought an essential element in the stabilization of complex technologies. For society to think knowledge and technology legitimate, then, neither can be decoupled from the values and norms in which they are produced and applied. In terms of co-production, the debate about prenatal diagnosis thus was a very necessary stage if this technology was to become part of the social order. Various actors—experts and representatives of different organizations—participated in the debate, which ranged over all the arguments about prenatal diagnosis, within the framework of key discourses that operated in accordance with their own logic and values.

In Sweden the debate about prenatal diagnosis did not lead to a change in the right to abortion. That right, like confidence in the woman's right to choose, was firmly rooted in the political discourse of the 1974 Abortion Act *and* in the medical discourse, and the practice of prenatal diagnosis was stabilized around these discourses. However, because of the official inquiries and discussions, there was a growing emphasis on the voluntary nature of prenatal diagnosis and the importance of women being given detailed, factual information, along with information about societal support to children with disabilities. Medical facts were not enough, information about prenatal diagnosis had to include its social and psychological aspects (Socialstyrelsen 1986). However, the highly charged and normative issues of the right and ability to choose foetal traits, would return in the following years as new medical knowledge and new technologies developed in genetics and reproductive medicine. The debate about prenatal diagnosis shows the importance of reflecting on this knowledge and its applications at an early stage. The social order it gives rise to will influence not only how the application of research is regulated, but also the conditions for future knowledge production.

Notes

1 This chapter was made possible by grant 2012–01048 from the Swedish Research Council for the project 'Better humans or reduced suffering? Historical perspectives on medical genetics and genetic counselling, 1950–1980'.

2 The eugenics movement was found in many parts of the world, see Bashford & Levine 2010.

3 The Sterilization Acts in force between 1935 and 1975 permitted sterilization without consent in certain situations. Roughly half of all sterilizations in the period were voluntary, but equally in half of cases there was coercion, pressure, or outright force. Coercion was most prevalent at the start of the period (SOU 2000:20).

4 The indications for abortion in the 1938 Act were medical, humanitarian, and eugenic. In 1946 a socio-medical indication was added, and in 1963 serious foetal defects.

5 The Swedish National Board of Health and Welfare was the government agency responsible for social services, public health, and the health service.

6 Riksarkivet (Swedish National Archives) (RA), Stockholm, Socialstyrelsens arkiv, SN2, Sjukhusbyrån, 5E1:191, Kjessler, Lindsten, Zetterström till Socialstyrelsen, 12 Jan. 1972.

7 In eighties culture, images of foetal development had been established as a genre of their own, largely because of Lennart Nilsson's acclaimed *Ett barn blir till* (1965, *A child is born*) which ran to several editions (Jülich 2015). It was launched as a book about foetal development and practical advice for pregnant women, but the complex issues of prenatal diagnosis, birth defects, and selective abortion were hardly mentioned—it was first published before the advent of prenatal diagnosis, and the second revised edition of 1976 referred to it in passing. Neither the right to an abortion nor selective abortion was mentioned. However, Nilsson's detailed colour photographs of the development of the foetus from fertilized egg to newborn baby contributed to the idea that the foetus had personhood. The images were in some contexts used to argue against late abortions in particular (Jülich 2017).

8 The motion was referred for consultation. Consultation responses were received from the National Medical Research Council, the Swedish Medical Society, the National Board of Health and Welfare, and the universities' medical and legal faculties. The Parliamentary Committee on Employment and Social Affairs recommended the motion be denied, and it was duly rejected by Parliament (Riksdagens protokoll 1972:127).

9 RA, Socialstyrelsens arkiv 1968–1981, SN1, Medicinalbyrån, E1:561c, Föreningen utvecklingsstörda barn (Association of Mentally Handicapped Children), Remissyttrande över Socialstyrelsens rapport *Fosterdiagnostik: Rapport från en av Socialstyrelsen tillsatt expertgrupp* 1982 (hereafter Remissyttrande).

10 RA, Socialstyrelsens arkiv, 1968–1981, SN1, Medicinalbyrån, E1:561c, Handikappförbundens centralkommitté (Swedish Disability Federation Central Committee), Remissyttrande.

11 RA, Socialstyrelsens arkiv 1968–1981, SN1, Medicinalbyrån, E1:561c, Synskadades Riksförbund (National Association for the Visually Impaired), Remissyttrande.

12 The synod brought together all the Swedish bishops of the Church of Sweden, the Lutheran state church.

13 Behind the report were Erwin Bischofberger DD SJ, Professor Holsten Fagerberg (Department of Theology, Uppsala University), Professor Gustav Giertz (Delegation for Medical Ethics, Swedish Medical Society), Sven Hemrin ThD, Professor

Jan Lindsten (Clinical Genetics, Karolinska University Hospital, Stockholm), and Anne-Marie Thunberg LTh.

14 RA, Socialstyrelsens arkiv 1968–1981, SN1, Medicinalbyrån, E1:561c, Föräldraföreningen för hjärt- och lungsjuka barn (Swedish Heart and Lung Association's Parents' Association), Remissyttrande.

15 RA, Socialstyrelsens arkiv 1968–1981, SN1, Medicinalbyrån, E1:561cRA, Socialstyrelsens arkiv 1968–1981, SN1, Medicinalbyrån, E1:561c, Svenska Läkaresällskapet (Swedish Medical Society), Remissyttrande.

16 RA, Socialstyrelsens arkiv 1968–1981, SN1, Medicinalbyrån, E1:561c, Svenska Läkarförbundet (Swedish Medical Association), Remissyttrande.

17 There had never been any question of screening all pregnant women using amniocentesis. However, AFP screening was trialled by taking blood samples from pregnant women in some health regions. The test was relatively simple and inexpensive, and indicated if the foetus had a neural tube defect. There was a degree of uncertainty concerning the test, though, and in some cases it had to be followed up with other tests such as amniocentesis.

18 RA, Socialstyrelsens arkiv 1968–1981, SN1, Medicinalbyrån, E1:561c, Föräldraföreningen för hjärt- och lungsjuka barn och ungdomar, Remissyttrande.

19 RA, Socialstyrelsens arkiv 1968–1981, SN1, Medicinalbyrån, E1:561c, De handikappades riksförbund (National Association of the Disabled), Remissyttrande.

20 When the National Board of Health and Welfare referred its report on prenatal diagnosis for consultation to a large number of organizations and government authorities, the women's associations were noticeable by their absence. However, after they complained they were added to the list of official consultation bodies.

21 RA, Socialstyrelsens arkiv 1968–1981, SN1, Medicinalbyrån, E1:561c, Sveriges socialdemokratiska kvinnoförbund (Sweden's Social Democratic Women's Association), Remissyttrande.

22 RA, Socialstyrelsens arkiv 1968–1981, SN1, Medicinalbyrån, E1:561c, Fredrika Bremerförbundet (Fredrika Bremer Association), Remissyttrande. The core mission of the non-partisan Fredrika Bremer Association, one of Sweden's oldest women's organizations, was gender equality.

23 RA, Socialstyrelsens arkiv 1968–1981, SN1, Medicinalbyrån, E1:561c, Vänsterpartiet kommunisternas kvinnopolitiska utskott (Left Party Communist Women's Political Committee), Remissyttrande.

24 RA, Socialstyrelsens arkiv 1968–1981, SN1, Medicinalbyrån, E1:561c, Kristen Demokratisk Samlings Kvinnoförbund (Christian Democratic Women's Association), Remissyttrande.

25 RA, Socialstyrelsens arkiv 1968–1981, SN1, Medicinalbyrån, E1:561c, Riksförbundet för Sexuell upplysning (Swedish Association for Sexuality Education), Remissyttrande.

26 RA, Socialstyrelsens arkiv 1968–1981, SN1, Medicinalbyrån, E1:561c, Svenska Läkarförbundet, Remissyttrande.

27 RA, Socialstyrelsens arkiv 1968–1981, SN1, Medicinalbyrån, E1:561c, Svenska Läkaresällskapet, Remissyttrande.

28 RA, Socialstyrelsens arkiv 1968–1981, SN1, Medicinalbyrån, E1:561c, Svenska läkaresällskapet, Humangenetiska sektionen (Swedish Medical Society, Human Genetics Section), Remissyttrande.

29 RA, Socialstyrelsens arkiv 1968–1981, SN1, Medicinalbyrån, E1:561c, Synskadades Riksförbund (Swedish Association of the Visually Impaired), Remissyttrande.

References

Åkerman, Henrik (1982), '1,2 miljarder per år i samhällsvinst möjlig med screening av alla gravida', *Läkartidningen*, 79, 2439–42.

Anér, Kerstin (1972), 'Angående individens okränkbarhet', Motion till Sveriges riksdag 1972:24 [motion in Swedish Parliament], https://data.riksdagen.se/fil/13A5DE53-C961-4A78-97DE-5B1A1028968F.

Bashford, Alison & Philippa Levine (2010) (eds.), *The Oxford handbook of the history of genetics* (New York: OUP).

—— (2010), 'Epilogue: Where did eugenics go?', in Bashford & Levine 2010, 539–58.

Björkman, Maria (2015), 'The Emergence of genetic counseling in Sweden: Examples from eugenics and medical genetics', *Science in context*, 28, 489–513.

—— & Anna Tunlid (2017), 'The establishment of genetic counselling in Sweden: 1940–1980', in Heike I. Petermann, Peter S. Harper & Susanne Doetz (eds.), *History of human genetics: Aspects of its development and global perspectives* (Cham: Springer International).

Broberg, Gunnar & Mattias Tydén (2005), 'Eugenics in Sweden: Efficient care', in Gunnar Broberg & Nils Roll-Hansen (eds.), *Eugenics and the welfare state: Sterilization policy in Denmark, Sweden, Norway, and Finland* (East Lansing: Michigan State University Press).

Comfort, Nathaniel (2012), *The science of human perfection: How genes became the heart of American medicine* (New Haven: Yale University Press).

Dagens Nyheter (10 June 1980), 'Fosterdiagnostik kan bara avslöja ärftliga sjukdomar'.

—— (17 June 1980), 'Fosterdiagnostikens problem: Kyrkan vill ha en etisk debatt'.

—— (18 June 1980), 'Fostertest: rätt eller plikt?'

—— (23 July 1982), 'Enhetliga regler behövs'.

—— (27 July 1982), 'Kritiker till fosterdiagnostik: Ekonomiskt tänkande skapar farlig moral'.

Ecks, S. (2008). 'Three propositions for an evidence-based medical anthropology.' *JRAI Supplement*: S77–S92.

Fagerberg, Holsten (1980), 'Inledning' in id. (ed.), *Foster, familj, samhälle: Fosterdiagnostikens innebörd och etik* (Lund: Liber Läromedel).

FUB-kontakt (1978), 'Det handlar om synen på människovärdet och samhället', 13(4), 2.

—— (1982), 'Fosterdiagnostik', 17(4), 14–15.

Giertz, Gustav (1980), 'Våra slutsatser', in Fagerberg, Holsten (1980) (ed.), *Foster, familj, samhälle: Fosterdiagnostikens innebörd och etik* (Lund: Liber Läromedel), 115–25.

Gustafson, Sture (1980), *Fosterdiagnostik för vem?* (Stockholm: LT).

—— (1984), *Vem har rätt att födas? En bok om människosyn och fosterdiagnostik* (Stockholm: LT).

Gustavson, Karl-Henrik (1967), 'Genetisk rådgivning ur pediatrisk synvinkel', *Läkartidningen*, 64, 3137–50.

—— (1978), 'Genetisk upplysning och prenatal diagnostik', *Läkartidningen*, 75, 2201–2202.

Hagberg, Bengt & Karl-Henrik Gustavson (1978), 'Prevention av psykisk utvecklingsstörning', *Läkartidningen*, 75, 415–16.

Harper, Peter S. (2006), 'The discovery of the human chromosome number in Lund, 1955–1956', *Human Genetics*, 119, 226–32.

Irwin, Alan, Torben Jensen & Kevin Jones (2013), 'The good, the bad and the perfect: Criticizing engagement practice', *Social Studies of Science*, 43(1), 118–35.

Jasanoff, Sheila (2004) (ed.), *States of knowledge: the co-production of science and the social order* (London: Routledge).

——(2005), *Designs on nature: Science and democracy in Europe and the United States* (Princeton: PUP).

Jülich, Solveig (2015), 'Lennart Nilsson's *A child is born*: The many lives of a best-selling pregnancy advice book', *Culture Unbound*, 7, 627–48.

—— (2017), 'Picturing abortion opposition in Sweden: Lennart Nilsson's early photographs of embryos and fetuses', *Social History of Medicine*, 31(2), 278–307.

Kevles, Daniel J. (1995), *In the name of eugenics: Genetics and the use of human heredity* (Cambridge, MA: Harvard University Press).

Kjessler, Berndt, J. Lindsten, R. Zetterström & P.-A. Ockerman (1972), 'Prenatal diagnostik av genetisk sjukdom', *Läkartidningen*, 69, 2362–3.

—— (1979), 'Vem har rätt att portionera ut lidande och ångest till de gravida och deras familjer?', *Läkartidningen*, 76, 1155–6.

Lambert, H. (2006). "Accounting for EBM: notions of evidence in medicine." *Soc Sci Med* 62(11): 2633-2645.

Lambert, H., E. J. Gordon, et al. (2006). 'Introduction: gift horse or Trojan horse? Social science perspectives on evidence-based health care.' *Soc Sci Med* 62(11): 2613–2620.

Lennerhed, Lena (2017), *Kvinnotrubbel: Abort i Sverige 1938–1974* (Möklinta: Gidlunds förlag).

Lindee, Susan (2005), *Moments of truth in genetic medicine* (Baltimore: Johns Hopkins University Press).

Lindsten, Jan, et al. (1975), 'Genetisk rådgivning i sjukvården: Etiska och psykologiska aspekter', *Nordisk Medicin*, 90, 71–8.

—— et al. (1976), *Klinisk genetik: Supplement till Medicinsk service* (Stockholm: Social-styrelsen).

Löwy, Ilana (2017), *Imperfect pregnancies: A history of birth defects and prenatal diagnosis* (Baltimore: John Hopkins University Press).

Melander, Stig (1978), 'Individen inom och utom livmodern', *Läkartidningen*, 75, 3281–4.

Nordlund, Roland, et al. (1978), 'Pengarna eller livet: En betraktelse över prenatal diag-nostik', *FUB-kontakt*, 13(2), 3–4.

Rose, Nikolas (2007), *The politics of life itself: Biomedicine, power, and subjectivity in the twenty-first century* (Princeton: PUP).

Socialstyrelsen (1982), *Fosterdiagnostik: Rapport från en av Socialstyrelsen tillsatt expert-grupp* (Stockholm: Socialstyrelsen).

—— (1986), *Fosterdiagnostik: Om att informera och stödja föräldrarna* (Stockholm: Socialstyrelsen).

SOU (Statens Offentliga Utredningar) (2000:20), *Steriliseringsfrågan i Sverige 1935–1975: Historisk belysning—Kartläggning—Intervjuer*.

Stockholms-Tidningen (5 July 1982), 'Missbrukad fosterdiagnostik ger fascistiskt samhälle'.

—— (22 Nov. 1982), 'Fosterdiagnostik på gott och ont'.

Svenska Dagbladet (17 Mar. 1971), 'Analys av fosterbarn minskar arvssjukdom'.

—— (9 Dec. 1979), 'Vid livets gräns'.

—— (18 June 1980), 'Den ofödda människan'.

Svenska Läkaresällskapets delegation för medicinsk etik (1979), 'Rätten till abort', in *Etiska värderingar—Medicinskt handlande* [1972] (Stockholm: Svenska Läkaresällskapet).

—— (1980), 'Etiska synpunkter på fosterdiagnostik [1979]', in Holsten Fagerberg (ed.), *Foster, familj, samhälle: Fosterdiagnostikens innebörd och etik* (Lund: Liber Läromedel).

Tydén, Mattias (2002), *Från politik till praktik: De svenska steriliseringslagarna* (Stockholm: Almqvist & Wiksell International).

Upsala Nya Tidning (17 June 1980), 'Utredningen om fosterdiagnostik: Vi måste få ny abortdebatt'.

Wahlström, Christina (1974), 'Vi skulle inte klara ett mongoloidbarn till', *FUB-kontakt*, 9(4), 14.

CHAPTER 2

The objects of global health policy

Turning knowledge into evidence at the World Health Organization

Rachel Irwin

In December 2012, I received a box with a picture of a mother and baby. It was a 'Nourishing newborns feeding kit', which, according to the text on the outside, included an 'easy-to-follow guide to breast and bottle feeding, valuable savings on infant formula and Similac savings for your baby'. The box also had the slogan, 'Newborns don't come with a feeding manual. But Similac® StrongMoms® does'. In addition to this box, between July 2011 and December 2012 Abbott Laboratories, the makers of Similac, sent me five direct mailings advertising Similac Infant Formula and each including a $5 coupon.

At the time, I was researching the UNICEF/WHO International Code of Marketing of Breastmilk Substitutes. The Code was adopted in 1981 in response to the unethical marketing of infant formula, especially in low-income settings. The direct mailings I received thirty years later were a violation of the Code, specifically Article 5 which prohibits both the direct advertising to mothers and coupons. I reported this to the International Baby Food Action Network (IBFAN), an international non-governmental organization (NGO). IBFAN relies on a grassroots network to supply it with examples of Code violations or inappropriate private sector involvement. As part of their work, they run the International Code Documentation Centre in Penang, Malaysia, to which people can report violations. The Centre responded, letting me know that they had received similar reports from mothers in Canada and the US. My complaint, and those of the mothers referenced in the letter, eventually fed into IBFAN reports, including updated versions of *Breaking the Rules, Stretching the Rules*, a biannual report produced by IBFAN that presents evidence on violations of the Code. IBFAN uses the report as an advocacy tool, for example using excerpts in flyers to hand out at WHO meetings with the aim of influencing policymakers.

This vignette describes how an object—or a photographic representation of it—can be transformed from a promotional tool, manufactured at an Abbott factory, into a piece of evidence which is then used in advocacy at the WHO in Geneva, Switzerland. In a broader sense, public health knowledge and experience are embedded in an object which is then used as evidence to inform policy.

Empirical and theoretical approaches

The transformation of public health knowledge and experience into evidence is fundamental to the work of the World Health Organization (WHO). As the United Nations' (UN) specialized agency for health, the WHO constitution mandates it to 'propose conventions, agreements and regulations, and make recommendations with respect to international health matters' and to 'develop, establish and promote international standards' in the health sector. In order to fulfil these core functions of 'setting norms and standards' in public health and 'articulating ethical and evidence-based policy options' (WHO 2019), the WHO also calls on experts to prepare independent and evidence-based reports. However, as a member state organization, the process of making recommendations and regulations also formally involves representatives from 194 countries, and often includes other UN bodies, civil society, and the private sector. A key question is how (or if) the WHO produces policies that are globally relevant through this process. How are public health knowledge, evidence, and experience from 194 member states and a wide range of other stakeholders incorporated into policies that are meant to be universally applicable?

I examine this question by comparing the production of two WHO policies: the *International Code of Marketing of Breastmilk Substitutes* (1981) and the *Set of Recommendations on the Marketing of Foods and Non-alcoholic Beverages to Children* (2010). The latter, developed in response to concern at increasing rates of childhood obesity, sets out ways for member states to 'reduce the impact on children of marketing of foods high in saturated fats, trans/fatty acids, free sugars, or salt.' In drafting both the Set of Recommendations and the Code, the WHO involved member states, experts, civil society, and the private sector in the shape of the food and pharmaceutical industries. Both documents were formally adopted and endorsed by WHO member states at the World Health Assembly (WHA), the WHO's main governing body.

Empirically, my comparison is based on interviews with key stakeholders behind both documents, ethnographic fieldwork at WHO headquarters in Geneva, archival material, and documentation from WHO governing body meetings. I interviewed 46 individuals, spanning WHO staff, staff from other relevant UN bodies, representatives from member states (including the WHA delegations), NGOs, and private industry (including advertising and the food and beverage sectors), and researchers involved in the case studies as experts. After the Set of Recommendations was endorsed by the WHA, the WHO was tasked with producing an implementation guide. This document sets out policy options and suggestions for incorporating the Set of Recommendations into national contexts. I carried out six months of participant observations at WHO headquarters, working in the team responsible for the Set of Recommendations and contributing to the writing of the implementation guide, which was finalized in 2012. In the course of the fieldwork, I came across information and experience embedded in many physical and digital objects—reports, flyers, peer-reviewed articles, systematic reviews, logos, products, and brands—which are the subjects of this chapter.

The policy process at the WHO revolves around the transformation of public health experience and knowledge into evidence. Such knowledge and experience often come in the form of systematic reviews of peer-reviewed literature, official recommendations by expert committees, and data on disease trends and burdens. In the case of the Code and the Set of Recommendations, evidence also includes documented violations of the Code or other marketing techniques considered inappropriate by the various actors in the case studies. Formal decisions, or resolutions, taken by the WHA, not only cite evidence, they also become evidence in that they can be cited in future resolutions. In fact, any object can become evidence when it is used to prove a point. In the policy context, evidence only exists in relation to a question (Engelke 2008). That is, knowledge and experience of the marketing of food or infant formula is organized into evidence depending on who is using it and for what purpose, and evidence must be *for* something (Engelke 2008). In other words, the Similac® kit was 'just' an object, but became evidence when used by breastfeeding advocates to prove that Abbott was violating the Code. In other words, as Åsa Alftberg notes in this volume, knowledge is mediated through material objects.

The narratives of these two case studies demonstrate how policymaking at the WHO is the result of the interaction among public health knowledge, evidence, emotion, and a range of situational, social, and environmental factors that influence political feasibility (Walt 1994, 29–33; Hodžić 2013). We also see that the global health community continues to struggle and experiment with ranking and using different types of evidence in creating policy. On the one hand, the superiority of evidence can be fetishized and used to create the illusion that policy stakeholders are morally superior and acting impartially according to what the evidence 'says'. In this way, the use of evidence can be a way to assert power. On the other hand, evidence is a social product whose truth can be challenged. Indeed, treating evidence as truth can obscure the subjective, ideological, and political nature of the production of evidence (Goldenberg 2006). For example, criticisms of randomized controlled trials (RCT) and evidence-based medicine focus on how these movements and tools have inappropriately quantified the social and political processes that interact with health, or have ignored them completely (Lambert 2006; Lambert et al. 2006; Goldenberg 2006; Ecks 2008). In another example in this volume, Kristofer Hansson, Gabriella Nilsson, and Irén Tiberg look at the challenges of implementing evidence-based care practices in real-life settings. Evidence can also be challenged on the basis that those who produce it are biased—as in both of the cases I mentioned at the start of this chapter.

Beyond this, the policy process at the WHO is characterized by both politics and aesthetics. Major policies, such as the Code or the Set of Recommendations, must be agreed upon by 194 member states. Each of these countries has their own social, cultural, and political contexts which influence how they vote or push for certain policy choices in Geneva. This also creates a situation in which powerful lobbies or advocacy groups at the national level can influence member states to make certain decisions at the WHO, and pressure other countries to do the same. At the same time, WHO documents represent a certain type of genre, and knowledge and evidence must be massaged so that it fits the aesthetic constraints of international policy documents (Hodžić 2013; for press releases, see Lindh in this volume).

In what follows I look at how public health knowledge and experience were transformed into evidence, which in turn was used to produce both the Code and the Set of Recommendations. In doing so, I consider the use of evidence for agenda-setting and as a rationale for action, controversies about evidence, and how the 'best available evidence' promotes or limits certain policy options.

Evidence as a rationale for action

I begin with breastmilk substitutes: at the 27th WHA in 1974, fifteen WHO member states sponsored a draft resolution that was adopted as Resolution WHA27.43. Its preamble stated:

> Reaffirming that breast-feeding has proved to be the most appropriate and successful nutritional solution for the harmonious development of the child; ... Noting the general decline in breast-feeding, related to sociocultural and environmental factors, including the mistaken idea caused by misleading sales promotion that breast-feeding is inferior to feeding with manufactured breast-milk substitute. (WHO 1974, 1)

This was the first mention in the WHO record of the issue of marketing of breastmilk substitutes, and it noted evidence and experiences of the decline in breastfeeding.[1] Less than ten years later, the WHO would adopt the International Code of Marketing of Breastmilk Substitutes. Here I will trace the history leading up to the adoption of the Code.

The decline of breastfeeding rates and the rise of commercial feeding had their origins in the industrial era and shifts in women's roles (Palmer 2009). Broadly, industrialization led to increased female employment outside the home in settings that were not conducive to breastfeeding. 'Scientific products' such as infant formula were promoted as 'modern' and 'better'. In the first half of the twentieth century, the increasing Westernization of medicine continued this trend, so that by the Second World War artificial feeding was promoted as the norm in much of the US and Europe (Post & Baer 1980; Palmer 2009; Allain 2005, 8). Other reasons cited for the decline in the mid twentieth century included a lack of education in general, lack of education about breastfeeding, family influences, working conditions, and healthcare practices (WHO 1981, 7, 14–24).

In the post-war period, companies also began to market their products heavily in low- and middle-income countries. According to the WHO, this marketing of breastmilk formula was a factor in the decline of breastfeeding:

> Another factor is the infant food industry. While it has met certain needs it has also diffused new and inappropriate ideas on infant feeding and has often created an unnecessary demand. The advertising and promotion of breast-milk substitutes, particularly in health facilities, may have contributed to the decline in breastfeeding. Promotion of breast-milk substitutes by commercial concerns has been more extensive and pervasive than provision of information about the advantages of breast-milk and breastfeeding. (WHO 1981, 17)

Companies marketed their products in ways that many NGOs and others working in health considered to be unethical. For instance, companies gave medical workers misleading literature and free samples, and, dressed in white coats, gave starter packs of formula to new mothers while still in hospital (Jelliffe 1971; Werner & Saunders 1997). This was not limited to low- and middle-income countries, but health workers and activists were particularly concerned about the promotion in poor resource settings.

Specifically, they were concerned by the misuse of infant formula, leading to higher infant mortality. This included mixing formula with contaminated water, diluting formula to make it last longer, or the use of non-appropriate foods as formula such as sweetened condensed milk (Werner & Saunders 1997). The difference in mortality between breastfed and formula-fed babies was noted as early as 1910 (Davis 1913). In the 1930s, Cecily Williams—later the first director of Maternal and Child Health at the WHO—warned of unsanitary, diluted breastmilk substitutes (Joseph 1981). In the 1950s and 1960s, doctors across Africa were 'dismayed by the numbers of younger infants suffering from the diarrhoea and malnutrition that came to be called "bottle-baby disease"' (Palmer 2009, 240). The issue here, as in Europe and the US at the turn of the century, was that much of the population did not have access to clean drinking water. Also, on account of poverty, mothers were diluting the formula to make it last longer, further contributing to malnutrition. An additional concern in poor resource settings was the high costs of treatment for ill babies (Post & Baer 1980).

The concern expressed by healthcare providers gained attention in the popular press in the early 1970s. The New Internationalist magazine published an interview with two paediatricians who had worked in Africa. Then in 1974, the British charity War on Want published *The Baby Killer*, which was infamously translated into German as 'Nestlé kills babies' (Palmer 2009, 242). Perhaps what garnered more attention was not the publication itself, but Nestlé's libel suit against War on Want (Chetley 1988).

By this time, religious groups were also concerned about the promotion of infant formula. The World Council of Churches' Christian Medical Commission addressed the issue in several of its newsletters (Barrow 1976).[2] In the US context, the Interfaith Center on Corporate Responsibility, a coalition of national church bodies and Roman Catholic orders, investigated the issue and, finding that many of its constituent national church bodies and Roman Catholic orders held shares in companies that sold infant formula, decided to encourage its membership to file shareholder resolutions. At first these resolutions were simply requests for information and clarification about marketing practice, but as marketing practices were documented in ever-greater detail they began to take legal action. For example, in 1976 the Sisters of the Precious Blood, who held shares in Bristol Myers, filed a lawsuit against them for misleading sales promotion. The Infant Formula Action Coalition grew out of these grassroots efforts to launch a boycott of Nestlé in 1977, which attracted a growing number of breastfeeding groups, such as Baby Milk Action in the UK.

The result was that the issue entered the political arena, where it was picked up by US Senator Edward Kennedy. He pursued it at both the national and the international level, even insisting that the WHO send a representative to testify to Congress and later requesting that the WHO organize a conference to consider the development of an international Code (McCoy 1995).[3] Prompted by Senator Kennedy's letter along with 'deep concern felt by many people, organizations and governments about the state of health and nutrition of the infant and young child' the WHO and UNICEF called a joint meeting in October 1979 (WHO 1981, 10). Experts and stakeholders discussed information about energy needs, normal weight gain, milk production and composition, anti-infective factors in human breastmilk, and mechanisms of prevention. They also considered information on trends in breastfeeding and its role in birth spacing (WHO 1981). The WHO had set up a collaborative study that ran between 1976 and 1978 to gather evidence on breastfeeding, specifically 'to define the current state of breastfeeding more clearly and to identify the factors contributing to change'. In it they studied 23,000 mother and child pairs from Chile, Ethiopia, Guatemala, Hungary, India, Nigeria, the Philippines, Sweden, and Zaire, countries chosen to represent broad regional, cultural, and socioeconomic differences across the WHO, with participants selected from a range of rural and urban locations and according to their socioeconomic status (WHO 1981, 130).

One recommendation to come out of this meeting was that 'there should be an international code of marketing of breast-milk substitutes' (WHO 1981, 10). Over the next two years, the WHO Secretariat consulted with member states, other UN agencies, NGOs and consumer groups, scientists, and the food industry. They went through several drafts of the International Code, which was revised following further consultation. The final version was endorsed by the 34th WHA in May 1981. It was widely seen as a success, with only the US voting against it and three other countries abstaining.

At the 34th WHA, delegates submitted interventions, citing evidence to argue for the Code. The Iranian delegate noted the health benefits of breastfeeding, stating that:

> Breastfeeding not only provided the child with a considerable amount of maternal antibodies, thus protecting it against communicable disease. It also created an emotional and psychological interdependence between mother and child which resulted in well-balanced physical and mental growth. (WHO 1982a, 11)

The delegates of Turkey and Canada, respectively, made similar points on the 'superiority' of breastmilk over infant formula, with Turkey arguing that 'no one questioned the superiority of breastmilk'.

> Indeed, the biological and psychological benefits of breastfeeding were so well established that it would be superfluous to elaborate on them, except perhaps to say that every year added more knowledge of breastmilk's unrivalled anti-infective and nutritive properties. (WHO 1982b, 3–4)

Canada said that 'the superiority of breastmilk—psychological, nutritionally, immunologically—was beyond dispute. Hence breastfeeding must be encouraged and produced as one of the measures essential to the vary [*sic*] survival of many infants and desirable for the health development of all the world's children' (WHO 1982b, 4).

The Code provides guidance on how companies may ethically market products to healthcare providers and to mothers, including, but not limited to, the following measures:

> All products should include clear labels with the benefits and superiority of breastmilk;
> Labels should also clearly state the hazards of improper preparation of breastmilk substitutes;
> No advertising of breast milk substitutes to the general public;
> No free samples to pregnant women, mothers or members of their families;
> No promotion in health care facilities, including no free supplies. (WHO & UNICEF 1981)

The WHO Code per se is non-enforceable, but many WHO member states have incorporated parts of it into their own national laws, which are in line with the Code (Allain 2005; Palmer 2009). Companies have subsequently been taken to court in several countries, either for false advertising or for breaking national law in member states. For example, in the mid-1990s a consumer group in India took Nestlé to court for violating the Infant Milk Substitutes, Feeding Bottles and Infant Foods (Regulation of Production, Supply and Distribution) Act 1992 (Jindal 1996; Bouckley 2012). Primary monitoring of the Code is carried out by a global network of breastfeeding groups, under the wider umbrella of the International Baby Food Action Network, and the reporting on the Code's implementation is typically discussed every other year at the WHA.

In the next section, I turn to the marketing of food and non-alcoholic beverages to children. In high-income countries childhood overweight and obesity levels began to rise in the 1980s, alongside a rise in adult levels. Obesity and overweight are multifactorial, with a number of causes and suggested reasons for the increase. At a micro level, these include levels of physical activity, parental eating habits, breastfeeding, and early child nutrition; at a macro level, both the academic and popular discourses have focused on the nutrition transition, including the role of modernization and industrialization in the food and agriculture sectors, the growth of transnational companies, and trade liberalization (Zimmet 2000; Hawkes 2007), and specifically the role of fast-food companies, agricultural subsidies, high fructose corn syrup, and the marketing of unhealthy food (Schlosser 2001; Nestle 2002). These dietary changes are not limited to high-income settings (Kennedy 2005; WHO 2010). In fact, low- and middle-income countries bear the greatest burden of diet-related non-communicable diseases (NCDs) (WHO 2011).

Philip James of the International Obesity Task Force was one of the first researchers to raise concerns about the specific role of the marketing of food and non-alcoholic beverages to children as a significant contributor to the rise in childhood obesity. The first milestone was his 1997 report to the UK government, *Healthy English schoolchildren: A new approach to physical activity and food* (James & McColl 1997), in which he discussed corporate promotion in schools. Two subsequent studies were also influential in setting out the evidence base, raising awareness of the issue, and contributing to national policy: the so-called 'Hastings Review', and an Institute of Medicine (US) study in 2006. Gerald Hastings and colleagues published the first systematic review of the effects of food promotion on children for the British Food Standards Authority (Hastings et al. 2003). Policy recommendations included restrictions on broadcast advertising and the sponsorship of products high in fat, salt, or sugar during and around programmes with a disproportionately high child audience. Three years later, the US Institute of Medicine produced the report, *Food Marketing to Children and Youth: Threat or Opportunity?* (IOM 2006).

During the first five decades of the WHO's existence, the organization, with a few notable exceptions, neglected non-communicable disease, focusing overwhelmingly on infectious disease. Those exceptions included a report by the WHO's Study Group on Diet, Nutrition and Prevention of Chronic Disease, published 1990. The WHO's first explicit recognition of the emerging obesity epidemic came in 2000 when it published a technical report on obesity, subtitled *Preventing and Managing the Global Epidemic* (WHO 2000). It was thus in the late 1990s that the WHO's work on food marketing began. 'Recognising the growing burden of NCDs and the fact that up to 80 per cent of heart disease, diabetes and stroke and over a third of cancers can be avoided by avoiding risk factors' (WHO 2008), in 2000 the 53rd WHA endorsed the Global Strategy for the Prevention and Control of Noncommunicable Diseases. The WHO's mandate for action on marketing food to children is ultimately derived from this document.

In a report prepared for the WHO, *Marketing Food to Children: The Global Regulatory Environment*, Corinna Hawkes (2004) focused on the processes that were very visible to the consumer, namely advertising and promotion. The report considered food marketing and promotion to include (but not to be limited to) broadcast advertising (television and radio), in-school marketing, corporate sponsorship, product placement, online and digital marketing, sales promotions, and packaging, including everything from supermarket specials on certain items to product placements in television programmes (Hawkes 2004). In the period leading up to the Set of Recommendations, the bulk of marketing of food and non-alcoholic beverages to children was on television, but the Internet, films, music, games, viral marketing, events sponsorship, and cross-promotions (such as toys in fast-food meals) were also notable sources (Harris et al. 2009).

The 60th WHA saw the passing of Resolution 60.23 on the Prevention and Control of Noncommunicable Disease: Implementation of the Global Strategy (WHO 2007), which asked the Director-General to use the Global Strategy for the Prevention and Control of Noncommunicable diseases as a basis for developing an action plan (WHO 2008). As part of Resolution WHA 60.23, the Director-General was asked 'to promote responsible marketing of foods and non-alcoholic beverages to children, in order to reduce the impact of food high in saturated fats, trans-fatty acids, free sugars, or salt, in dialogue with all relevant stakeholders, including private-sector partiers, while ensuring avoidance of potential conflict of interest.' It also called upon the WHO Secretariat to develop a set of 'recommendations on marketing of foods and non-alcoholic beverages to children' (WHO 2007).

As part of the process of drafting the Set of Recommendations, Hastings and his colleagues were asked to write two reports for the WHO on global data. In 2009, the WHO published their study, *The extent, nature, and effects of food promotion to children*, in which they reviewed studies from the 1970s up to 2008. Although the data was mixed, overall they found that food promotion did indeed influence food preferences, preferences for branded over unbranded products, and purchase-related behaviour (Cairns et al. 2009; Hastings et al. 2003; Livingstone 2005). The WHO

Secretariat convened an ad hoc expert group on food marketing for a week-long meeting to look at the evidence base for policy recommendations, including Hastings and his colleagues' reports. The WHO also consulted with member states and held two sets of stakeholder dialogues in Geneva with the private sector and NGOs respectively (WHO 2012).

At the 63rd WHA in 2010, the WHO Secretariat presented its recommendations on the marketing of food and beverages to children, as mandated by Resolution 60.23. They were duly passed as Resolution 63.14. The recommendations present a range of policy options for member states and, although much of the onus falls on them to implement the marketing policies—whether as government regulations, private sector voluntary pledges, or a combination—the WHO can offer assistance in developing policies if wished. One form this took was the 2012 implementation guide for the Set of Recommendations, a document that provides national and regional policymakers with concrete options for implementing the Set of Recommendations.

In the foreword to the Set of Recommendations, Dr Ala Alwan, then Assistant Director-General for Noncommunicable Disease and Mental Health, cites evidence of the global burden of obesity and overweight among children and its effects:

> Overweight and obesity now ranks as the fifth leading risk for death globally. It is estimated that in 2010 more than 42 million children under the age of five years are overweight or obese, of whom nearly 35 million are living in developing countries. Overweight during childhood and adolescence is associated not only with an increased risk of adult obesity and NCDs, but also with a number of immediate health-related problems, such as hypertension and insulin resistance. (WHO 2010, 4)

He then points to the role of marketing in childhood obesity:

> But at the same time, the wide availability and heavy marketing of
> many of these products, and especially those with a high content
> of fat, sugar or salt, challenge efforts to eat healthily and maintain
> a healthy weight, particularly in children. (WHO 2010, 4)

Although he does not cite any specific studies of marketing, this is inferred, and he does refer to the overall process, which included an analysis of such studies. With his statement that 'The recommendations were developed with substantial input from Member States and other stakeholders and endorsed by the Sixty-Third World Health Assembly in May 2010' (WHO 2010), he implies that member states' and other stakeholders' experiences were indeed incorporated into the final document.

In both case studies it is clear that evidence and experience were the precursors to serious international action. The ad hoc expert group and academics both noted that 'evidence was a given' and that the Set of Recommendations 'couldn't have happened without the evidence—like Gerald Hasting's work', pointing to the importance of research.

Once a health issue reaches the WHO, evidence provides the justification for action and confers on it the necessary 'moral authority'. By invoking evidence, actors give the impression they are acting rationally to improve health and well-being. Although policymaking at the WHO is situated in wider social, political, and economic contexts, the use of evidence in these interventions was a key depoliticizing strategy. This is seen in the statements by the Turkish, Canadian, and Iranian delegates at the 34th WHA: by invoking evidence, it makes diplomats seem as if they are 'above' politics and acting impartially, even as they gloss over the wider context of the situation and the political nature of evidence (Goldenberg 2006).

A key difference between the making of the Code and the Set of Recommendations was that the Code relied far more on expert opinion and stakeholder views, particularly at the 1979 Joint WHO/ UNICEF meeting and in the drafting process. This was highlighted by a report published by the WHO in 1981, based on the paper prepared for the 1979 Joint WHO/UNICEF meeting. While not meant to be a 'scientific treatise', it nevertheless set out to 'stimulate further thought and discussion' among 'national-level health workers and planners' (WHO 1981, 12); it did include such statements as 'several studies indicate that breastfed infants have fewer gastrointestinal infections than those not breastfed' (WHO 1981, 109), but provided no references.

Today, greater transparency in the way evidence is collected and analysed is expected, and this transition has been seen at the WHO. Before 2007, WHO recommendations were based largely on expert opinion and did not use 'systematic evidence-based methods'. Public criticism of this process led the WHO to develop a Guidelines Review Committee (GRC) to standardize the process and assert a level of quality control (Sinclair et al. 2013). In a study led by the clinical researcher David Sinclair, eighteen WHO staff were interviewed about their experience of the GRC. Overall, the interviewees felt that it was essential to the WHO that its guidelines met the highest standards; however, some had concerns about the way in which the GRC takes a single approach to ranking types of evidence, for instance prioritizing randomized controlled trials over observational studies. The concern is that this may work very well for clinical guidelines, but may be less appropriate for health systems or public health guidance.

With the Set of Recommendations, the WHO spelt out very clearly how its systematic reviews were conducted, and gave references and summaries for all the studies reviewed, which are publicly available (Cairns et al. 2009). These reviews are also cited in the final Set of Recommendations. Overall, in line with the move towards evidence-based medicine, the WHO has increasingly taken a more systematic, evidence-based approach to policymaking. In this case, however, the evidence linking childhood obesity to food marketing is not conclusive. This has proved to be fertile ground for controversy.

Controversies about evidence

It is difficult to link the marketing of food directly to childhood obesity. In the systematic reviews commissioned by the WHO, 115 studies met the criteria for inclusion, of which only 46 were 'capable of demonstrating a potential causal relationship between food promotion and children's food knowledge, preference and behavior' (Cairns et al. 2009, 10). The remaining studies were content analyses of advertisements or other type of promotions, or they were surveys of food consumption or purchasing behaviour, or rather children's purchase requests to their parents. There are natural experiments as marketing aimed at children has been highly restricted in Norway, Sweden, and Quebec since the 1980s, but the evidence as to the usefulness of such bans is mixed (Kent et al. 2011). Still, marketing remains an 'easy' policy choice in that it is 'legislable'.

In interviews with private sector informants, representatives from the food industry discussed the mixed nature of the evidence. For instance, one stated that

> I would say in general, that there is no sure cause-effect relation between advertising and obesity … obesity is definitely a multi-factorial phenomenon. For example, most families have two cars … causes range from transport to health to culture. Yes, advertising is a part. But a part.

Another complained about 'academic activists' publishing headline-grabbing studies that are based on 'bogus' evidence—or at the very least, evidence that had been manipulated or presented in what they saw as an anti-industry way. The same informant also felt that that NGOs have greater influence at the WHO. Specifically, he suggested that many academics have a political bias which 'taints' their work, yet because many of them work closely with the WHO—in expert groups, collaborating centres, and as consultants—their academic work is affected by their politics. He went on to explain the main obstacle to the food industry producing evidence, namely that it is virtually impossible to publish any industry-funded research in academic journals, although he felt like this was beginning to change.

Almost all civil society informants, meanwhile, compared the food industry to the tobacco industry, citing the way that private sector actors 'deny, deflect or diffuse' public health evidence. One, who had worked closely with the WHO, discussed 'dismissal, denial, acceptance and pre-emption'. These strategies range from industry representatives who dismiss the quality of evidence to companies which, accepting the 'unhealthiness' of their food, introduce new 'healthy' ranges of popular products. It also includes companies that focus on multiple causes of obesity or on lack of physical activity as a cause (rather than diet).

Broadly speaking, the evidence as collected, analysed, and presented by academics working for the WHO is mixed. Many private sector actors use this to shift the focus away from their unhealthy products—a tactic that is part of the wider quest for legitimacy. By creating doubt, the private sector delegitimizes its critics; when the evidence is stronger, the private sector must participate in partnerships with government or other regulatory processes if it is to maintain its legitimacy (Benson & Kirsch 2010).

The controversies and dilution of the evidence about breastfeeding are similar. A representative from an infant formula company pointed out that the decline in breastfeeding was multifactorial, citing issues with maternity leave and ease of pumping that have nothing to do with her company's production of food. Indeed, although delegates at the WHA in 1981 asserted that the 'superiority of breastmilk was beyond dispute', the reality is that there were—and remain—conflicts about evidence. For example, in September 1981 the editor-in-chief of *Pediatrics* wrote:

> Picture yourself, a doctor living in a Third World country frustrated by the failure of your efforts to change poverty, malnutrition, and poor sanitation. Little wonder that you would choose to attack rich foreign companies if you thought they contributed

to your problems. You would also feel great if the whole world joined you in condemning such companies. When the turmoil had settled, however, and you realized that you may have been wrong, or at least lacked proper evidence, you might not feel so self-righteous. (Lucey 1981, 431)

The evidence to limit the marketing of breastmilk substitutes was not strong in the way we expect evidence to be strong today. Much of the evidence for the Code was based on the experiences of health professionals working in low-income countries. If the Code were written today the evidence *for* it would be expected to come from systematic reviews and quantitative, replicable studies. And yet, despite all the research in the nearly forty years since the Code, the issue has not been settled. In the 1980s and 1990s, evidence on breastfeeding was called into question because of concerns about HIV transmission between mother and child (Newell 2001). Other researchers have questioned the WHO/ UNICEF recommendations of exclusive breastfeeding for six months (rather than four months), suggesting that new systematic reviews were needed. This was in part due to concerns about the higher incidence of food allergies and risk of coeliac disease among breastfed children (Fewtrell 2011).

There is a performative aspect to evidence (Ecks 2008, S85). This means that an individual, say a clinician, may use the same study or statistic differently depending on the audience, patient, colleague, or academic journal. When scaled up to a global level, we see that policymaking at the WHO involves people who use the same body of evidence to forward the agendas of their country or organization. While the underlying knowledge and experiences may be the same, they are used to created different sets of evidence depending on the situation.

This is particularly the case with both the Code and the Set of Recommendations, in which the evidence base is mixed. Most global health actors would suggest that the move towards standardization and evidence-based policymaking is a positive step. There is also the suggestion that it lends greater legitimacy and authority to guidelines, as in the case of the Sinclair et al. study (2013). However, it also raises the question of what policymakers should do when the evidence is not clear, as is often the case in situations of international concern. I discuss this in the next section.

Evidence and policy options

The way evidence is used both constricts and expands the possible policy options. With the Set of Recommendations, the WHO convened an ad hoc expert group who were asked to 'Provide technical advice in three areas':

> Policy objectives: What should be the objectives of Member States policies on marketing of food and non-alcoholic beverages to children;
> Policy options: What are the evidence-based or currently applied policy options available on marketing of foods and nonalcoholic beverages to children;
> Monitoring and evaluation: What are the feasibility and mechanisms required to monitor and evaluate recommended policy options. (WHO 2012, 1)

The groups focused on the responsibilities of the various stakeholders, the range of policy recommendations and options (statutory versus non-statutory), the age ranges of the children, and where protection from marketing pressure was needed.

A 2012 special issue of *The Economist* argued that food companies influenced the Set of Recommendations, which led to watered-down, general recommendations:

> Food companies are among those that present their view to the WHO … through the WHO's 'public dialogue' process. For example, companies encouraged the WHO to present a menu

of possible policies on food marketing, rather than a single prescription. (*The Economist* 2012)

Another point of contention has been the role of voluntary measures, including self-regulation (Sharma et al. 2010). Since 2006, individual companies and industry-wide bodies have made a series of voluntary promises to restrict the types of foods marketed and the venues and modes of advertising. For example, this might include ceasing to use cartoon characters to promote foods, or not promoting foods with an 'unhealthy' nutritional profile to children. Critics argue that voluntary self-regulation is ineffective, in part because the ways in which companies define foods as healthy or not healthy is not transparent or uniform across countries or regions. Also, there are virtually no examples of self-regulation being effective (Moodie et al. 2013). The Set of Recommendations leave open the possibility of self-regulation, in part because at the time there was not the evidence to rule it out completely. Research has since been published indicating that self-regulation pledges are too limited and inconsistent to be effective, and that the private sector has not followed through on wider promises to self-regulate (Hawkes & Harris 2011; Kraak et al. 2016).

I find the criticisms that industry influenced the Set of Recom-
mendations somewhat misleading. One problem is the lack of direct evidence. According to an informant from the expert group, they 'thought critically of the evidence and their duty and respon-
sibility' to be independent. This same informant said that 'there was no evidence for the interventions, which is part of the reason we couldn't make concrete recommendations'. A second member of the expert group also noted that they 'knew the evidence base wasn't there to fully rule out self-regulation.' I also specifically asked informants from the ad hoc expert group whether the private sector had influenced the Set of Recommendations, to which one responded that 'I would not use the word influence, but there was the recognition that we needed to provide a range of options and recognize reality.' Similarly, another said there was 'indirect

influence because we knew the political reality, attitudes [...] and this shaped the direction and frame of recommendations.' The same informant pointed out that they had consulted the reports from the private sector and civil society dialogues, and in that sense they were aware of the range of possibilities that were politically feasible. Another believed that the WHO Secretariat had suggested Corinna Hawkes as the chair of the ad hoc expert group because she 'knew the political possibilities.' Companies and the way they interact with governments and public health actors—through various types of partnerships and platforms—help determine the policymaking environment, and thus the options open to policymakers.

A concept that was often discussed during my participant observation at the WHO was the precautionary principle. Known from other civil society and member state fora, this is the idea that 'the introduction of a new product or process whose ultimate effects are disputed or unknown should be resisted' (OED 2013). Applied to food marketing, the precautionary principle would suggest that policymakers should restrict the marketing of foods high in fats, salt, and sugar to children unless food companies can prove it has no ill effect on child health. The food policy expert Amandine Garde, who has worked as a consultant to the WHO, writes that:

> while there is at present no conclusive scientific evidence that controls on food advertising directed at children alone are likely to lead to direct reductions in either consumption or harm, there is evidence that the promotion of food impacts on cultural attitudes and patterns of eating. An absence of conclusive evidence should not be interpreted as evidence of an absence of any adverse effect. (Garde 2006, 15)

The point here is that sometimes there is a justification—perhaps a moral justification—for making policy in the lack of direct and conclusive evidence.

Another challenge which impacted on the final Set of Recommendations was the reliance on studies from high-income countries. The WHO ad hoc expert group considered two systematic reviews of *The extent, nature, and effects of food promotion to children* (Cairns et al. 2009, Hastings et al. 2007), the more recent (led by Georgina Cairns) being an update of the first. A total of 115 studies met the inclusion criteria, of which only 10 studies had a component on countries outside Europe, the US, Canada, Australia, or New Zealand, 6 focused on a middle-income country, and only 2 were carried out in a low-income country (Nepal and Solomon Islands). This lack of input from low- and middle-income countries was also found in the countries and organizations represented in the stakeholder dialogues, few of whom had experience of low- or middle-income countries. The authors of the studies were well aware of the limitations and tried to mitigate them: in the first review, researchers conducted supplemental desk research using the business and marketing press, journals and responses from NGOs to map the marketing environment in low- and middle-income countries (Cairns et al. 2009,18); in the later review, there is an entire section devoted to 'food promotion and marketing in developing and middle-income countries' which teases out more detailed data from the 10 applicable studies. Additionally, there was geographic diversity in the ad hoc expert group.

While global representation is a goal at the WHO, there are few health issues that are evenly distributed across the globe. Georgina Cairns and colleagues found that food companies in middle-income countries used marketing techniques similar to those in high-income countries at the time, but had very little data on low-income settings. This meant that in the final version of the Set of Recommendations there was greater focus on television and online advertising and less on advertising methods in low-income countries at the time, such as billboard, print, and point-of-sale.

One informant, an academic who had worked closely with the WHO, discussed the difference between evidence-based and evidence-informed policy, suggesting that 'good policy should not be solely evidence-driven'—that is, sometimes the evidence is non-existent, not strong enough, or not in the right form to justify policy action, but that due consideration of the evidence which does exist and some common sense can justify policy action. Generally speaking, the quality or type of evidence can either constrict or expand policy options. A lack of clear evidence also decides the policy options. If the Code were developed today, it would need to be supported by more developed evidence than was available at the time. Evidence, however, interacts with emotion and political feasibility, which means that decisions can be pushed forward in the absence of evidence.

Where knowledge and experience become evidence

Both the Code and the Set of Recommendations embody a narrative of how groupings of actors—diplomats, WHO staff, academic experts, civil society and private sector actors—brought a range of ideas, beliefs, values, and experiences to the drafting process. In both cases, civil society actors and health professionals used their knowledge and experience, mediated through objects, to put inappropriate marketing on the WHO's agenda; they continue to work to keep it there, for example by collecting data on violations of the Code nearly 40 years later. The WHO's role in all this is to gather and then turn public health knowledge and experience into evidence, which, in turn, is used to determine policy. This often means assembling expert groups and commissioning systematic reviews. Stakeholders use evidence and moral arguments to justify to donors and other policymakers why action should be taken to address the underlying causes of various health problems. Addressing global inequities in health is a justification for global health action (Rosskam & Kickbusch 2012, 4).

Delegates to the WHA use persuasive language and descriptions of the health burdens in their countries. Words like 'urge' are used to propose action. Evidence is also used as a tool to assert moral legitimacy and as a depoliticizing strategy. If actors 'have the evidence on their side' they can push for certain policy options over others. Yet some views are simply not taken into account. This is a source of contention for anthropologists such as Judith Justice, who have focused on the applicability of global norms to communities (Justice 1987). The national-level civil servants who sign up to agreements in Geneva are not the same people who survey supermarkets for inappropriate marketing practices. Although the Code and Set of Recommendations are ostensibly global documents, the impetus for the Code originated in the marketing situation faced by low- and middle-income countries, while the Set of Recommendations grew out of the situation in high- and upper-middle-income countries.

There have always been disagreements over the quality and interpretation of evidence. One change, however, is that in comparing the Code to the Set of Recommendations the global health community expects more methodologically robust evidence today. It also expects greater transparency about what kind of knowledge and experience is used as evidence in decision-making. The negotiation and scope of solutions are now more dependent on the robustness of the evidence than they were in the 1970s and 1980s. On the one hand, this is democratizing, for when evidence and decision-making is more transparent, a wider range of actors is informed about and can participate in the policy process. On the other hand, if the evidence is inconclusive and if actors are averse to the precautionary principle, then the interests of consumer industries may prevail and public health action may be constrained.

Writing of co-production, Sheila Jasanoff notes that 'what we know about the world is intimately linked to our sense of what we can do about it, as well as to the felt legitimacy of specific actors, instruments and course of action' (2004, 14). The case studies considered here highlight the wider context of policy-making and constraints on action, and the ways in which power is embedded in the sense of reality. For instance, in the case of the Set of Recommendations the expert committee took into account the 'reality' of a global society in which transnational companies wield significant influence over regulators. There is also an aesthetic element to the process: knowledge and experience must be presented in certain ways to become evidence. Similarly, actors are expected to behave according to culture scripts in order to be 'successful' in legitimizing their experience and knowledge as evidence, and actors can be criticized for deviating from the script, for example by acting emotionally. These case studies challenge any notion that evidence is apolitical, demonstrating instead the flexible arrangements found in the transformation of experience and knowledge into evidence for policy-making.

Notes

1　Starting in the late 1960s, the UN Protein Advisory Group, which included the WHO, began to discuss concerns about bottle feeding.
2　The Christian Medical Commission was disbanded in the 1990s, but the World Council of Churches remains an active NGO in official relations with the WHO (Litsios 2004, 1892).
3　WHO Archives, Edward Kennedy to Halfdan Mahler, 20 July 1978.

References

Allain, Annelies (2005), *Fighting an old battle in a new world* (Uppsala: Dag Hammarskjöld Foundation).

Barrow, Ruth Nita (1976), 'Breast feeding—A myth or a must?', *Contact Magazine* [Geneva, World Council of Churches], 2–5.

Benson, Peter & Stuart Kirsch (2010), 'Capitalism and the politics of resignation', *Current Anthropology*, 51(4), 459–86.

Bouckley, Ben (2012), 'Nestlé India faces charge for alleged infant formula labelling law violations', *Dairy Reporter*, 19 March.

Cairns, Georgina, Kathryn Angus & Gerard Hastings (2009), *The extent, nature and effects of food promotion to children: A review of the evidence to December 2008* (Geneva: WHO).

Chetley, Andrew (1988), *The politics of baby foods: The successful challenges to an international marketing strategy* (London: Pinter).

Davis, William H. (1913), 'Statistical comparison of the mortality of breastfed and bottle-fed infants', *American Journal of Diseases in Childhood*, 3, 234–47.

Ecks, S. (2008). 'Three propositions for an evidence-based medical anthropology.' *JRAI Supplement*, S77–S92.

Engelke, Matthew (2008), 'The objects of evidence', *Journal of the Royal Anthropological Institute*, S1–S21.

Fewtrell, Mary S. (2011), 'The evidence for public health recommendations on infant feeding', *Early Human Development*, 87(11), 715–21.

Garde, Amandine (2006), 'The regulation of food advertising and obesity prevention: What role for the European Union?' (EUI Working Paper 2006/16, Department of Law, European University Institute).

Goldenberg, Maya. J. (2006), 'On evidence and evidence-based medicine: Lessons from the philosophy of science', *Social Science & Medicine*, 62, 2621–32.

Harris, Jennifer L., Jennifer L. Pomeranz, Tim Lobstein & Kelly D. Brownell (2009), 'A crisis in the marketplace: How food marketing contributes to childhood obesity and what can be done?', *American Review of Public Health*, 30, 211–25.

Hastings, Gerard, Martine Stead, Laura McDermott, Alasdair Forsyth, Anne Marie Mackintosh, Mike Rayner, Christine Ann Godfrey, Martin Caraher & Kathryn Angus (2003), *A review of research on the effects of food promotion to children* (Glasgow: Centre for Social Marketing, University of Strathclyde).

—— Laura McDermott, Kathryn Angus, Martine Stead & Stephen Thomson (2007), *The extent, nature and effects of food promotion to children: A review of the evidence* (Geneva: WHO).

Hawkes, Corinna (2004), *Marketing food to children: The global regulatory environment* (Geneva: WHO).

—— (2007), *Globalization, food and nutrition transitions* (Geneva: Commission on Social Determinants of Health, WHO).

—— & Jennifer L. Harris (2011), 'An analysis of the content of food industry pledges on marketing to children', *Public Health Nutrition*, 14(8), 1403–14.

Hodžić, Saida (2013), 'Ascertaining deadly harms: Aesthetics and politics of global evidence', *Cultural Anthropology*, 28(1), 86–109.

IOM (US Institute of Medicine) (2006), *Food marketing to children and youth: Threat or opportunity* (Washington, DC: Institute of Medicine).

James, Philip & Karen A. McColl (1997), *Healthy English schoolchildren: A new approach to physical activity and food* (Aberdeen, Rowett Research Institute).

Jasanoff, Sheila (2004), *States of knowledge: The co-production of science and the social order* (London: Routledge).

Jelliffe, Derrick B. (1971), 'Commerciogenic malnutrition?', *Nutrition Reviews*, 30(9),199-205.

Jindal, Tarsem (1996), 'New developments in Nestlé court case in India' [letter to the editor], *BMJ*, 313, 1399.

Joseph, Stephen C. (1981), 'The anatomy of the infant formula controversy', *American Journal of Diseases of Children*, 135(10), 889–92.

Justice, Judith (1987), 'The bureaucratic context of international health: A social scientist's view', *Social Science & Medicine*, 25(12), 1301–1306.

Kennedy, Eileen T. (2005), 'The global face of nutrition: What can governments and industry do?', *Journal of Nutrition*, 135(4), 913–15.

Kent, Monique Potvin, Lise Dubois & Alissa Wanless (2011), 'Food marketing on children's television in two different policy environments', *International Journal of Pediatric Obesity*, 6, e433–e441.

Kraak, Vivica I., Stefanie Vandevijvere, Gary Sacks, Hannah Brinsden, Corinna Hawkes, Simón Barquera, Tim Lobstein & Boyd A. Swinburn (2016), 'Progress achieved in restricting the marketing of high-fat, sugary and salty food and beverage products to children', *Bulletin of the WHO*, 94(7), 540–8.

Lambert, H. (2006). 'Accounting for EBM: Notions of evidence in medicine.' *Soc Sci Med* 62(11): 2633–2645.

Lambert, H., E. J. Gordon, et al. (2006). 'Introduction: Gift horse or Trojan horse? Social science perspectives on evidence-based health care.' *Soc Sci Med* 62(11): 2613–2620.

Livingstone, Sonia (2005), 'Assessing the research base for the policy debate over the effects of food advertising to children', *International Journal of Advertising*, 24(3), 273–96.

Lucey, Jerold F. (1981), Editor's note, *Pediatrics*, 68, 431.

McCoy, Charles, (1995), *Case 6: Nestlé and the controversy over the marketing of breast milk substitutes* (Columbus, OH: Council for Ethics in Economics).

Moodie, Rob, David Stuckler, Carlos Monteiro, Nick Sheron, Bruce Neal, Thaksaphon Thamarangsi, Paul Lincoln & Sally Casswell [*The Lancet* NCD Action Group] (2013), 'Profits and pandemics: Prevention of harmful effects of tobacco, alcohol, and ultra-processed food and drink industries', *The Lancet*, 381, 670–9.

Nestle, Marion (2002), *Food politics* (Berkeley & Los Angeles: University of California Press).

Newell, Mary-Louise (2001), 'Prevention of mother-to-child transmission of HIV: Challenges for the current decade', *Bulletin of the WHO*, 79(12).

OED (2013), *Oxford English Dictionary*, s.v. 'precautionary principle', oxforddictionaries.com.

Palmer, Gabrielle (2009), *The politics of breastfeeding: When breasts are bad for business* (London: Pinter & Martin).

Post, James E. & Edward Baer (1980), 'The international code of marketing of breastmilk substitutes: Consensus, compromise and conflict in the infant formula controversy', *International Commission of Jurists Review*, 25, 52–6.

Rosskam, Ellen & Ilona Kickbusch (2012) (eds.), *Negotiating and navigating global health: Case studies in global health diplomacy* (New Jersey: World Scientific Publishing).

Schlosser, Eric. (2001), *Fast food nation: The dark side of the all-american meal* (Boston: Houghton Mifflin).

Sharma, Lisa L., Stephen P. Teret & Kelly D. Brownell (2010), 'The food industry and self-regulation: Standards to promote success and to avoid public health failures', *American Journal of Public Health*, 100(2), 240–6.

Sinclair, David, Rachel Isba, Tamara Kredo, Babalwa Zani, Helen Smith & Paul Garner (2013), 'World health organization guideline development: An evaluation', *PLoS ONE*, 8(5), e63715.

The Economist (15 Dec. 2012), 'Special report: Obesity'.

Walt, Gill (1994), *Health policy: An introduction to process and power* (Johannesburg: Witwatersand University Press).

Werner, David & David Sanders (1997), *Questioning the solution: The politics of primary health care and child survival* (Palo Alto: HealthWrights).

WHO (1974), *Infant nutrition and breast-feeding* (Resolution WHA27.43; Geneva: WHO).

—— (1981), *Infant and young child feeding: Current issues* (Geneva: WHO).

—— & UNICEF (1981) *International code of marketing of breastmilk substitutes* (Geneva: WHO).

—— (1982a), *Summary records from the 13th meeting of Committee A of the 34rd World Health Assembly* (Geneva: WHO).

—— (1982b), *Summary records from the 14th meeting of Committee A of the 34rd World Health Assembly* (Geneva: WHO).

—— (2000), *Obesity: Preventing and managing the gobal epidemic* (Report of a WHO Consultation, WHO Technical Report Series; Geneva: WHO).

—— (2007), *Prevention and control of non-communicable diseases: Implementation of the global strategy* (Resolution WHA60.2; Geneva: WHO).

—— (2008), *2008–2013 Action plan for the global strategy for the prevention and control of noncommunicable diseases* (Geneva: WHO).

—— (2010), *The set of recommendations on the marketing of foods and non-alcoholic beverages to children* (Geneva: WHO).

—— (2012), *Process for the development of a set of recommendation on the marketing of foods and non-alcoholic beverages to children* (Geneva: WHO).

—— (2019), 'About WHO', http://www.who.int/about/role/en/.

Zimmet, Paul (2000), 'Globalization, coca-colonization and the chronic disease epidemic: Can the doomsday scenario be averted?', *Journal of Internal Medicine*, 247, 301–310.

PART II

CIRCULATING AND SHARING

MEDICAL KNOWLEDGE

CHAPTER 3

Sharing knowledge

Neuroscience and the circulation of medical knowledge

Åsa Alftberg

Knowledge has long been studied in the social sciences and the humanities with focus on its production and construction. For example, Science and technology studies (STS) has explored and revealed the making of scientific knowledge in particular contexts, often the lab, and the ordering of science and knowledge has been linked to the ordering of society (Jasanoff 2004). As Sheila Jasanoff (2004) has stated, doing science is related to power and merges into doing politics. The making of science is a history of knowledge dependent on power and culture. In Jasanoff's words, science and society are co-produced, each underwriting the other's existence.

A complementary but different approach which has gained traction recently is the *circulation* of knowledge. The concept directs attention towards 'how knowledge moves, and how it is continuously moulded in the process' (Östling et al. 2018, 17). For Johan Östling and his colleagues, inspired by work by the likes of Philipp Sarasin and Andreas Kilcher, the circulation of knowledge is characterized by the mediality and materiality of knowledge (18). Knowledge is embedded in social contexts and for the most part mediated through material objects. It is always formed by power relations and cultural processes, which implies that the accessibility of knowledge is dependent on its specific position, time, and place, and differs between societies. As it circulates, knowledge—like notions, things, people—often transforms (Markovits et al. 2006). The circulation of knowledge is profoundly affected by digitalization, as communication—infrastructure and content, production and circulation—has changed. The changed conditions for the circulation of knowledge have an impact on the forms and exercise of power (Couldry 2012). Digitalization can strengthen some forms of power and weaken others, just as it strengthens some forms of knowledge (legitimizing them so they are taken as given) and lessens others.

In this chapter, medical knowledge and its circulation is explored using an example from neuroscientific research, where neuroscientists in focus-group interviews talk about sharing knowledge in different contexts. Sharing knowledge is here identified as a form of knowledge circulation. Sharing knowledge is about spreading information, moving it from one context to another, and the process is permeated with different layers of intentions, interpretations, and meaning-making. As part of a wider circulation, sharing knowledge as a concept highlights the intentional and interactive aspects of the process. I will describe different aspects of sharing knowledge, as they are discussed by researchers in the field of medical knowledge. The medical knowledge in question is the specialized field of neuroscience that is engaged in the search for potential cures for neurodegenerative diseases, so in other words part of a larger paradigm of the medical knowledge frequently examined by the medical humanities.

By exploring views on medical knowledge and its circulation from the perspective of a privileged group—the scientists who are the main actors in producing medical knowledge—the complexity of knowledge circulation can be emphasized. Following James Secord (2004), I consider how and why knowledge circulates, and what happens when it ceases to be the exclusive property of a single individual or group and becomes part of the tacit knowledge held by much wider groups of people.

Interviews as sharing knowledge

The empirical material of this chapter consists of qualitative focus-group interviews with neuroscientists at a university in southern Sweden. The interviews were carried out in a research project about the various framings of the human brain that influence neuroscientific work, and the connection to wider cultural interpretations of the brain.[1] In the focus-group interviews, participants were asked to describe their work and laboratory procedures. The focus was on their perceptions, opinions, beliefs, and attitudes concerning their work, and sharing knowledge was an aspect that came up in the interviews. The participants were members of two research groups that work with neurons in a laboratory environment, looking for treatments for neurodegenerative diseases. Four focus-group interviews of one to one and a half hours' duration with 3–5 participants apiece were conducted between November 2015 and May 2016. The interviews were transcribed verbatim, but material is presented here with anonymized names and research projects.

Focus-group interviews can themselves be regarded as a form of knowledge-sharing, as they are conversations that produce, share, and circulate knowledge between participants, not just between participants and interviewer. This process is of course influenced by the questions raised and the nature of the interaction between the participants, as there is always the possibility that the participants will direct their attention towards agreement rather than acknowledging differences (Gray 2003). In the present case this will probably have been lessened by the fact that the participants were colleagues who knew one another well.

Another important aspect is that interviews, by dint of being transcribed, become texts. The shared knowledge from the interviews is interpreted, reread, and sorted into patterns by the researcher. A written text can be scrutinized in a way that a verbal conversation cannot. It also vests in the researcher—the interpreter—the power and prerogative of its content (Gunnemark 2011).

Knowledge circulation and neuroscience

The concept of circulation can be used as a theoretical perspective. According to Katja Valaskivi and Johanna Sumiala, it is the dynamic structures of circulation that are of interest, and how they connect to power:

> The simplest way of thinking about circulation is to say that it is about 'going around' and/or 'passing on' something—whether it is material or immaterial items, goods, artefacts, ideas or beliefs that are being distributed and disseminated. … In this circulatory process, certain ideas, items and actors become more powerful, while others may fade away or change their shape or consistency, thus taking other directions and creating new processes in circulation. (Valaskivi & Sumiala 2014, 231)

Valaskivi and Sumiala continue by describing three approaches to the topic of circulation. The first is to acknowledge circulation as a non-static, non-linear concept. They underline flexibility in the sense of the direction and tempo of movement. The second approach is to stress circulation as 'an open-ended process, a movement that brings ideas, items and people together' (233). This relates to action, and is explained as 'typically shaped by tensions, contradictions and ambiguities that are represented, reproduced and sustained in the circulation process' (233). Here, power relations shape circulation, but may simultaneously be contested. The third approach is that the materiality of circulation constitutes an essential aspect: circulation involves material objects, which are embedded in ideas, beliefs, ideologies, and emotions.

When such theories of circulation are applied to the circulation of medical knowledge it is easy to see how knowledge moves through academia and societies in a non-linear way (see Latour 1999; Raj 2007). The circulation of knowledge is driven by tensions, contradictions, and ambiguities, where power and resources give some actors better access—and greater credibility—than others.

The materiality of knowledge circulation is always present, for circulation relies on material objects (from research instruments and printed publications to online publications and information, such as lectures easily accessible through computers and mobile phones), which in turn affect the circulation process.

Another important aspect of medical knowledge circulation is that it is often scientific property. The knowledge is owned. And that ownership has consequences for the circulation process. Stephen Hilgartner (2004) explains that property is not simply things that are owned, but a bundle of rights connected to these entities, with specified limits. To possess property is to be embedded in a fabric of rights and obligations. Property may not always be explicitly recognized by the legal system, as in the example of scientific property, because the relevant property in scientific exchange includes not only formally recognized intellectual property (such as patents, copyrights, and trade secrets), but also what Hilgartner calls 'informal' types of scientific property, such as rights and obligations of the parties to a research collaboration or the authors of a scientific paper. Therefore, property as a concept, legally and morally, is linked to power relations. It is also deeply involved in scientific practices, and, as I discuss in this chapter, in medical knowledge circulation.

Neuroscience is a useful illustration of medical knowledge circulation. Current developments in brain research, with new technological and therapeutic possibilities, have transformed how we understand, manage, and treat people, amounting to an emerging neuro-ontology (Rose & Abi-Rached 2013; Hansson & Idvall 2017). The human condition is primarily understood as a self consisting of brainhood rather than personhood (Vidal 2009): people are cerebral subjects. As such, we have access to neuroscientific vocabulary and techniques, especially the colourful images of brain scans, as well as the common-sense notion that being human is exclusively physical and reliant on the brain (Zivkovic 2015). Knowledge of the brain circulates between neuroscience and the public, the media, and politics. It permeates popular culture: media products such as sci-fi series and films draw on neuroscience to build imagined, but still vaguely realistic, depictions of what new technology can do to the brain and, by extension, to people. Knowledge circulates back to academia, where neuroscientists are confronted with these (often distorted) representations when meeting patients, watching television, or describing their work to friends or the general public (see Hansson 2017a). The upshot is that the supposed distinction between science and popular culture is constantly challenged by the circulation of knowledge (Alftberg & Bengtsen 2018).

In the following, I will explore the circulation of medical knowledge and its power dimensions using empirical examples from a neuroscientific setting. I examine the concept of knowledge-sharing in the light of competition, collaboration, and problematic sharing—the themes which emerge when scrutinizing the empirical material for patterns and relevant thematics.

Competition

When the participating neuroscientists discuss their work in the interviews, it is clear that the aim of each of their research projects is to gain new knowledge. Research is described as a competitive game with projects that need to be innovative but not too risky. According to the participants, any research project has risks—for instance, will it be possible to develop new knowledge or not? If the risks are too great the project risks coming to a dead-end (see Hansson 2017b; Hammarfelt et al. 2016). A project that does not reach any new conclusions is considered a failure. Consequently, risk features in every project, but is connected to power factors such as influence and funding (which projects receive resources, who the influential researchers are, and so on). Academic careers are built on competition—competition for funding, for leadership, for impact, for international reputation (Müller 2014)—which also means there is always a risk of failure.

Medical knowledge, as we have seen, is looked on as property, belonging to one or several researchers, and this too fuels and is fuelled by the competitive nature of academia. Competition generates the risk of 'being scooped', when other researchers publish similar findings before you do, or of your idea being stolen. This is described by Daniel and Karen:

> Daniel: On the X-project I think it was very clear when we stated that this was a low-risk project based on the techniques, because we had everything set up and available. But it was clearly a high-risk project based on the competition, so we knew very well that it had to be done quickly. The high risk was that we knew that other researchers were about to do the same thing.
> Karen: Yes, the risk of being scooped.

Working on a research project and generating new results is a competition against time and other scientists, and there is always the risk that 'your' findings will be pre-empted by someone else. Knowledge is viewed as property that needs to be guarded and kept safe, an approach that hinders the circulation of medical knowledge. It is only once research findings are published that they are free to circulate and be shared. In other words, once medical knowledge is validated and has a clear ownership, sharing is possible. Nevertheless, as the participants explain, the reality is that ideas and knowledge sometimes are scooped, to be used and further developed by other researchers. Circulated, in other words.

The participants see a moral dilemma in doing an experiment that they know others are doing too. They note that, quite apart from the idea of knowledge as property (and property should be respected), on a societal level it could be regarded as a waste of taxpayers' money and, in the long run, reduced public confidence in science. On the other hand, there can be good reasons to do the same experiments, as Karen and Thomas discuss:

> Karen: But I think sometimes it's also a problem that people don't want to do the same as other people did because it's already published, and then you, you lack the validation and there's lots

and lots of data out there that hasn't been validated. And that's a big problem.

Thomas: It depends also on how clever one group versus the other puts that testing. And sometimes one group can be the first, but the other one makes it in a much cleverer way, and in a much more robust way.

Validating knowledge, and doing 'robust' tests to produce it, is a typical description of what is called evidence-based knowledge. Evidence-based knowledge is the process of systematically finding, appraising, and using contemporaneous research findings as the basis for rational decisions (Rosenberg & Donald 1995; Persson et al. 2017). Originating in medical science, evidence-based knowledge and practice have spread, for instance to social work, and today is the kind of scientific knowledge that commands particularly high confidence in academia and society (see Hansson, Nilsson & Tiberg and Irwin in this volume). It is considered first-rate knowledge with apparently objective verifications of what reality looks like.[2] As such, this is the kind of medical knowledge that the participants value, and, considering its high status, knowledge that ought to be circulated and shared.

Collaboration

While competition in science is discussed by participants, they dwell even more on the question of collaboration. Collaboration is associated with sharing knowledge. The participants reflect on how technological advances have opened the possibility of sharing:

Thomas: In science I consider competition not so useful as collaboration I'd say.

Karen: I guess people share more too.

Emma: Yeah, they share and it's more international.

Anna: It's possible to share. […] There's access to information and there are possibilities… technical possibilities for sharing.

Karen: Yeah, it's possible, it's part of technology. But it's also that, it becomes more common that the big labs, when they have a new technique they can… the more software and things… they just put it open source on the Internet, and people are free to use it. Instead of charging money for it or keeping it secret. I mean that's why the CRISPR, for instance this CRISPR technology of editing the human genes, one reason it's become so popular is because the people who developed it they put out software online or on their webpage, which makes it easy for other people to do the same.[3] To use the technique. So they shared that with everyone. So, I think it's a way of spreading your research to others.

Emma: It feels like in the last ten years that there is much, it gets much better every year. Like, from my point of view for the last ten years that view has changed a lot, you share much more and you've more commercially available tools for your research now than there were eight years ago or ten years ago.

It is not a new insight that technology and digitalization have changed the circulation of knowledge, but it is interesting to see how the participants reflect on the changes that have happened only in the last decade. It has altered their working conditions, but also their view on medical knowledge, and sharing is now 'natural'. Digitalization and the accompanying quantitative, metric-based measurability and the changes it has effected in working conditions in academia have been explored by Ruth Müller (2014), who highlights the experience of being in a highly competitive race that requires a continuously accelerating working pace as well as a strong focus on individual achievement. This relates to the concept of the 'entrepreneurial self' (Bröckling 2005), suggesting continuous self-improvement and flexibility, adapting to market needs (Müller 2014). On the other hand, as the quotes illustrate, digitalization and online availability can also lead to increased transparency and collaboration.

Technology and digitalization are not abstract phenomena, but are dependent on material objects. The materiality of knowledge circulation—the physical objects needed to produce and share it—affects the circulation (how, when, and how fast), and partially erodes the view of knowledge as property. In current research, sharing and collaboration could be more relevant than competition and keeping things to yourself (Laudel 2001; Müller 2012). Still, the reason for sharing should not be perceived as merely altruistic; sharing knowledge is a strategy for a successful career:

> Karen: I think today it [sharing] is viewed as a strategy for success. Whereas maybe previously it's been more like keeping secret. But today it's viewed as a route to success of actually sharing because that means that more people will cite your work and… […] It increases their impact.
> Anna: Because now it is possible to monitor the number of times that published works are cited…

The materiality of knowledge circulation has changed the conditions of scientific publication and publication rates. This in turn seemingly influences the way success is being defined: it is to be published and, even more importantly, to be cited (Hammarfelt 2017). Sharing may promote collaboration, but paradoxically, because of its connection to a successful career, it also promotes competition (see Müller 2014). According to the participants, the greater circulation of medical knowledge is a desired process. Nevertheless, there is also the underlying notion of 'the entrepreneurial self' (Bröckling 2005), where sharing knowledge in publications and the number of citations is a career strategy.

Problematic sharing

The participants also discussed how knowledge is shared between patients. For instance, patients may share (often positive) experiences of treatments and information they have acquired. This information is part of a medical circulation of knowledge outside academia, often using social media. Online social networking has changed how people communicate with one another, and how they identify relevant information and share it (Eysenbach 2008). One example is communication between people based on their medical diagnoses, creating patient forums where they can express and compare their experiences (see Hagen 2012). In the social media, patients' experiences may become ostensibly medical knowledge:

> Anna: Of course there's always people who feel that they are helped by this, then they do… advertise you know that 'I went there and it was great or I did that', on Facebook, which is a new way of communicating all sorts of things.
> Karen: It's easier to read Facebook than a scientific article.
> Anna: Yeah. And people hear what they want to hear. So if they want to feel better, they hear someone who felt better and they want to do the same thing. They don't want to hear the arguments why it wouldn't feel better.
> Thomas: And some of them actually cite scientific papers.
> Karen: Oh yes, really bad examples.
> Thomas: Twisted! They select a particular phrase and then they go bananas and just claim that… […] and there's no relationship.

This form of knowledge-sharing is regarded as problematic by the participants, since, according to them, the patients risk getting the information wrong or the wrong kind of medical knowledge. Even though there could be so-called expert patients with considerable knowledge about their diseases and new treatments, the participants feel that this only can instil false hopes of treatments or cures (for patient involvement, see Idvall in this volume).[4]

There is a global circulation of medical knowledge, which the sociologist and medical anthropologist Mary-Jo DelVecchio Good (2010) calls the medical imaginary. The medical imaginary—the affective and imaginative dimensions of biomedicine and biotechnology that embrace clinics, patients, and publics—circulates through professional and popular culture. Alternative stories, misuses, and failures of medicine's power and possibilities are also part of the medical imaginary (failures, fraud, discouragement, and greed); yet, broadly speaking it is an optimistic story of hope and the possibilities of medical science (Brown & Michael 2003). When patients share, access, and use this medical knowledge, it may be perceived as problematic though. According to the participants, the patients' sharing of information has its ethical risks and misunderstandings of what medical science can and cannot do. But there also seems to be an element of losing control. The scientists do not have control over the information that circulates in the social media. Again, referring to the idea of knowledge as a property, the implicit view is that medical knowledge belongs to science and the scientists, not the patients. Digitalization, such as social media, makes it more difficult to hold on to this distinction. However, the solution to the perceived lack of control is not to hinder information; rather it is to increase the distribution of correct medical knowledge (for example, by using social media), and to do so through being more active and engaged as a researcher. As one explains:

> Anna: What you can do is things like you can be active and present your research to the community. If you show alternatives, if you try to reach as many people as possible and you try to show that we are making progress at the universities, at the established research institutes, and then try to inform… Because I think that often they feel that nothing is going to happen at the universities for ten years, so I can't sit around and wait for that, I'll go elsewhere. If you try to describe the progress and things better…

Were people and patients to understand the ongoing knowledge production and progress in established research, they would not be tempted to 'go elsewhere' as Anna put it. According to the participants, patients desperate for new treatments are open to exploitation by commercial interests. Nancy Scheper-Hughes (2003) explains how advanced medical procedures and biotechnologies are now becoming part of new markets. The field of organ transplant is the most distinctive outcome of the combination of capital and medical technology in a transnational space, but there are also treatments that involve other body parts: tissues, cells, and reproductive and genetic material of others (Lundin 2012, 2015). When the participants discuss treatment 'elsewhere', they highlight how private clinics may offer medical treatments that are not tested and not safe for humans:

> Karen: There's a very big clinic in Ukraine, which is probably one of the biggest.
> Emma: Yeah, it was on the news today that they had transplanted a retina. That was not supposed to be in experiments, in pre-clinical research. But they had transplanted them into patients.

Another example is the use of stem cell transplants, where the participants draw a distinct line between their own research and clinical trials, and false treatments that are considered experiments with no scientific (for which read evidence-based) basis:

> Andrew: I think it's crazy that those places where you can do those stem cell transplants, that they even exist and that they're allowed to exist… fooling patients into believing they can be cured. That's really doing experiments on humans.
> Karen: There's no scientific background.
> Thomas: They will not say cure but will help this and that, and that's been going on in Europe and in the States because there is no regulation for that. You don't have to prove anything. You just have to… I think, I only think you need to show that, don't die from it, that's it. Otherwise, if it makes an improvement, no one cares.

Treatments that are not evidence-based or tested in clinical trials, with no requirement of proof, are not regarded as proper science. For the participants, going straight from findings in the lab to treatment, leaving out the trial stage, poses great risks to patients, and distinguishes this as a highly unethical and non-scientific procedure.

The circulation of medical knowledge is perceived as a misuse in cases like this. Also, commercial interests are contrasted to what science is and should be by definition, which becomes clear when Anna comments that the clinics' intention is not to cure people but to make money:

> Anna: It's just charging people money. It's not for advancing science, it's for making money… Because if they collected data from it, it would perhaps be somewhat helpful.

According to Anna, these experimental treatments might be useful if they were to collect the data involved, as the clinics would thus share their knowledge and contribute to the knowledge circulating about stem cell research. This contradicts the idea that there is no scientific basis to this; rather, if the clinics were to follow correct scientific procedure and produce evidence-based knowledge they *could* contribute. This ambivalence recurs in the discussion of these kinds of clinics. Participants agree, for example, that staff at these clinics are 'technically' researchers, because they have doctorates. As Anna says, 'Well I'm sure that they employ people with PhDs and MDs. And then they're technically researchers.' As such, they may even be encountered at scientific conferences:

> Karen: I met one of them [at a conference]. She came up to me and said how do you do that transplantation, do you just inject the cells in the blood? After talking to her it was really, really clear that they have… they don't know anything, they have no clue. They have no clue what they're doing.

Commercial clinic staff are not regarded as proper scientists and therefore sharing knowledge with them is impossible. Even though the clinic may have legal permission to obtain human embryos and have consent from the patients, the ethical aspects are too problematic. Karen says that she spoke her mind to the woman: they should not be doing anything like this at the clinic, and it could be a huge danger to the patients. Discussing the topic further, it appears that the physical risk to patients may not always be severe (even though it is never completely risk-free). It depends, for example, on whether the treatment involves injections of stem cells into the blood (injecting systemically) or into the brain:

> Anna: It's a lot cheaper to inject systemically than into the brain, it's a lot easier so… The risk is much lower than if you were to inject into the brain.
> Karen: Yeah. The most likely scenario is nothing will happen.

Accordingly, the physical risks to patients are often low (the patients' emotional turmoil, cast between despair and hope, and their financial investment in the treatment are other risks). Still, sharing knowledge in the situation described above is unimaginable, however low the risk to patients. Medical knowledge circulation has its limits, and the actors who produce knowledge can try to make it inaccessible for ethical and professional reasons.

The frictions of sharing knowledge

This chapter has explored the circulation of medical knowledge in a neuroscientific setting. It has illustrated situations where knowledge-sharing is considered by the participants to be useful and valuable, and situations when it is regarded as disadvantageous or highly problematic for ethical reasons.

The participants connect sharing medical knowledge to both competition and collaboration as well as a career strategy. There is an underlying aspect of power and influence: whose findings are spread and accepted, and how fast can it be done (in order not to get scooped)? The circulation of knowledge is affected by digitalization, which has changed the conditions of scientific publication and publication rates, and, by extension, success. It also creates tensions and contradictions. Sharing is both natural and expected, but you simultaneously risk 'your' knowledge being poached by someone else. Parallel to that, medical knowledge has to warrant the label of evidence-based if both academia and society are to hold it in high confidence.

Permeating the empirical examples is the idea that medical knowledge has ownership. It can be shared but it is always owned by someone, or by some more than others, and is part of power relations. The idea of property can be linked to the commodification of knowledge.[5] Medical knowledge as a commodity means that it should be valued by, and of service to, the market. It ought to be measured and controlled, just like any other resource. But, since the circulation of knowledge is non-static, non-linear, and flexible in its sense of direction and speed of movement, it defies control and produces what I have called problematic sharing. When sharing knowledge, it can rarely stay the exclusive property of a single individual or group. Rather, it becomes part of the accepted understanding of much wider groups of people, which may lead to criticism and disapproval from the group who see it as their property. Power relations are contested, as seen here in the use of digital media. According to the empirical examples, one strategy when knowledge (the property) is circulated and used in problematic, misinformed ways (as by patients) is to share information increasingly, and make sure it is the correct kind of medical knowledge that circulates (evidence-based). As one of the participants said, contributing accurate knowledge could bring patients to realize that treatments at commercial clinics are not an alternative. Another strategy is not to share knowledge at all, as in the example of encountering representatives of the commercial clinics at a scientific conference. The ethical risks involved for patients who are exploited by commercial clinics that offer non-evidence-based treatments are of course real, and should not be overlooked or downplayed. Nonetheless, ethical risks may well be used as arguments in order to guard and preserve the ownership of scientific knowledge, withholding power and privileged status.

To conclude, sharing medical knowledge is a process of intention and interaction, competition and collaboration. The concept of knowledge-sharing helps highlight how knowledge circulation is affected by digitalization, which changes scientific working conditions and sometimes makes sharing problematic. It reveals the underlying idea that knowledge is exclusive property, and the frictions that occur when this idea is challenged.

Notes

1 The project was financed by the Basal Ganglia Disorders Linnaeus Consortium and named 'What makes us human? Cultural perspectives on framings of the brain in neurological research'. The focus-group interviews were conducted by Kristofer Hansson, Markus Idvall, and Ellen Suneson.

2 At the same time, evidence-based knowledge is under fire from scientific disciplines founded on other epistemological grounds. The philosopher Maya Goldenberg (2006) points out that the seemingly unproblematic nature of evidence-based knowledge may be contested by emphasizing science as a social system of knowledge production. Evidence-based knowledge does not increase objectivity; rather it obscures the subjective elements that inevitably are part of all forms of human inquiry.

3 CRISPR is a family of DNA sequences in bacteria and archaea. It is a kind of molecular machinery designed to destroy intrusive DNA sequences, for example from viruses. It is used as a technology to affect DNA segments in the cell nucleus.

4 The expert patient (*spetspatient* in Swedish) is a patient who uses the Internet as an important source of disease-specific knowledge, and joins forces with fellow patients in patient organisations and similar. Riggare et al. 2017 describes this as an ongoing change for chronic conditions in healthcare: a shift from a model where healthcare professionals are experts and the patients are passive recipients of care to a model where patients are active participants who have the possibility to be experts in managing their own disease and situation. This indicates a reliance on patients' self-management and patient education, which can be problematized with the concept of self-care (see, for example, Hansson elsewhere in this volume; Alftberg & Hansson 2012).

5 This has long been a subject of discussion, for example Gibbons & Wittrock 1985; Gibbons et al. 1994; McKelvey & Holmén 2009; Benner & Widmalm 2011.

References

Alftberg, Åsa & Kristofer Hansson (2012), 'Introduction: Self-care translated into practice', *Culture Unbound: Journal of Current Cultural Research*, 4, 415–24.

—— & Peter Bengtsen (2018), 'The sci-fi brain: Narratives in neuroscience and popular culture', *Culture Unbound: Journal of Current Cultural Research*, 10(1), 11–30.

Benner, Mats & Sven Widmalm (2011), *Kunskap* (Malmö: Liber).

Bröckling, Ulrich (2005), 'Gendering the enterprising self', *Distinktion: Scandinavian Journal of Social Theory*, 6(2), 7–25.

Brown, Nik & Mike Michael (2003), 'A sociology of expectations: Retrospecting, prospects and prospecting retrospects', *Technology analysis & strategic management*, 15(1), 3–18.

Couldry, Nick (2012), *Media, society, world: Social theory and digital media practice* (Cambridge: Polity).

DelVecchio Good, Mary-Jo (2010), 'The medical imaginary and the biotechnical embrace: Subjective experiences of clinical scientists and patients', in, Byron J. Good, Michael M. J. Fischer, Sarah S. Willen & Mary-Jo DelVecchio Good (eds.), *A reader in medical anthropology: Theoretical trajectories, emergent realities* (Oxford: Wiley-Blackwell).

Eysenbach, Gunther (2008), 'Medicine 2.0: Social networking, collaboration, participation, apomediation, and openness', *Journal of Medical Internet Research*, 10(3), e22.

Gibbons, Michael & Björn Wittrock (1985) (eds.), *Science as a commodity: Threats to the open community of scholars* (London: Longman).

Gibbons, Michael, Camille Limoges, Helga Nowotny, Simon Schwartzman, Peter Scott & Martin Trow (1994), *The new production of knowledge* (London: Sage).

Goldenberg, Maya J. (2006), 'On evidence and evidence-based medicine: Lessons from the philosophy of science' *Social Science & Medicine*, 62, 2621–32.

Gray, Ann (2003), *Research practice for cultural studies: Ethnographic methods and lived cultures* (London: Sage).

Gunnemark, Kerstin (2011) (ed.), *Etnografiska hållplatser: Om metodprocesser och reflexivitet* (Lund: Studentlitteratur).

Hagen, Niclas (2012), 'A molecular body in a digital society', in Max Liljefors, Susanne Lundin & Andrea Wiszmeg (eds.), *The atomized body* (Lund: Nordic Academic Press).

Hammarfelt, Björn, Sarah de Rijcke & Alexander D. Rushforth (2016), 'Quantified academic selves: The gamification of research through social networking services', *Information Research*, 21(2).

—— (2017), 'Recognition and reward in the academy', *Aslib Journal of Information Management*, 69(5), 607–623.

Hansson, Kristofer & Markus Idvall (2017) (eds.), *Interpreting the brain in society: Cultural reflections on neuroscientific practices* (Lund: Arkiv Förlag).

—— (2017a) 'Mixed emotions in the laboratory: When scientific knowledge confronts everyday knowledge', in Hansson & Idvall 2017.

—— (2017b), 'Det mätbara arbetslivet i laboratoriet', *Kulturella Perspektiv*, 3–4, 8–17.

Hilgartner, Stephen (2004), 'Mapping systems and moral order: Constituting property in genome laboratories', in Sheila Jasanoff (ed.), *States of knowledge: The co-production of science and social order* (New York: Routledge).

Jasanoff, Sheila (2004), 'Ordering knowledge, ordering society', in ead. (ed.), *States of knowledge: The co-production of science and social order* (New York: Routledge).

Latour, Bruno (1999), *Pandora's hope: Chapters on the reality of science studies* (Cambridge, MA: Harvard University Press).

Laudel, Grit (2001), 'Collaboration, creativity and rewards: Why and how scientists collaborate', *International Journal of Technology Management*, 22(7–8), 762–81.

Lundin, Susanne (2012), 'Moral accounting: Ethics and praxis in biomedical research', in Max Liljefors, Susanne Lundin & Andrea Wiszmeg (eds.), *The atomized body* (Lund: Nordic Academic Press).

—— (2015), *Organs for sale: An ethnographic examination of the international organ trade* (London: Palgrave Macmillan).

Markovits, Claude, Jacques Pouchepadass & Sanjay Subrahmanyam (2006) (eds.), *Society and circulation: Mobile people and itinerant cultures in South Asia, 1750–1950* (London: Anthem).

McKelvey, Maureen & Magnus Holmén (2009) (eds.), *Learning to compete in European universities: From social institution to knowledge business* (Cheltenham: Edward Elgar).

Müller, Ruth (2012), 'Collaborating in life science research groups: The question of authorship', *Higher education policy*, 25(3), 289–311.

—— (2014), 'Racing for what? Anticipation and acceleration in the work and career practices of academic life science postdocs', *Forum: Qualitative Social Research*, 15(3).

Östling, Johan, David Larsson Heidenblad, Erling Sandmo, Anna Nilsson Hammar & Kari H. Nordberg (2018), 'The history of knowledge and the circulation of knowledge: An introduction', in eaed. (eds.), *Circulation of knowledge: Explorations in the history of knowledge* (Lund: Nordic Academic Press).

Persson, Johannes, Niklas Vareman, Annika Wallin, Lena Wahlberg & Nils-Eric Sahlin (2019), 'Science and proven experience: A Swedish variety of evidence-based medicine and a way to better risk analysis?', *Journal of Risk Research*, 22(7), 833-843.

Raj, Kapil (2007), *Relocating modern science: Circulation and the construction of knowledge in South Asia and Europe, 1650–1900* (Houndmills: Palgrave Macmillan).

Riggare, Sara, Pär J. Höglund, Helena Hvitfeldt Forsberg, Elena Eftimovska, Per Svenningsson & Maria Hägglund (2017), 'Patients are doing it for themselves: A survey on disease-specific knowledge acquisition among people with Parkinson's disease in Sweden', *Health Informatics Journal*, 1–15.

Rose, Nikolas & Joelle M. Abi-Rached (2013), *Neuro: The new brain sciences and the management of the mind* (Princeton: PUP).

Rosenberg, William & Anna Donald (1995), 'Evidence based medicine: An approach to clinical problem-solving', *BMJ*, 310, 1122–6.

Scheper-Hughes, Nancy (2003), 'Rotten trade: Millennial capitalism, human values and global justice in organs trafficking', *Journal of Human Rights*, 2(2), 197–226.

Valaskivi, Katja & Johanna Sumiala (2014), 'Circulating social imaginaries: Theoretical and methodological reflections', *European Journal of Cultural Studies*, 17(3), 229–43.

Vidal, Fernando (2009), 'Brainhood, anthropological figure of modernity', *History of the Human Sciences*, 22(1), 5–36.

Zivkovic, Marko (2015), 'Brain culture: Neuroscience and popular media', *Interdisciplinary Science Review*, 40(4), 409–417.

CHAPTER 4

Press releases as medical knowledge

Making news and identification in medical research communication

Karolina Lindh

Medical knowledge about the brain is not confined to labs, clinics, or the neuroscientific community. Neuroscientific research about the brain has gained explanatory value for many challenges that confront contemporary society and humans today. The increased public interest in this medical knowledge is noticeable in the publication of popular science books about neuroscience in recent years (for example, Aamodt & Wang 2008; Damasio 1994; Seth & Frith 2014). Another way in which medical knowledge about neuroscience circulates to reach wider audiences is in the shape of press releases. These briefly describe the results of studies, and commonly they also address what consequences the particular study may have for future treatments. In a scholarly setting, the publication of a paper implies that findings are made public (Borgman 2007, 48). This way in which findings are made public does however not necessarily mean they are easily accessible or comprehensible by people with no medical training. The writing of press releases, published in a variety of ways and actively promoted by university public relations officers, is designed to make findings available to the general public. The distribution of a press release may lead to a number of events, and publicity for the university or individual researchers if it catches the attention of news media. Although scholarly journal articles and scientific press releases may report findings from the same study, the ways in which this is done in these two genres is very different.

The business of translating the content of peer-reviewed journal articles into press releases intended for wider audiences than the scientific community often involves communication professionals. This group of professionals has grown in size at universities and academic institutions in recent decades, and has come to play an important role in representing their universities and the research done there to external audiences (for example, Hansson 2005). This work may involve a variety of activities and forms of science communication, among which the writing and distribution of press releases is one. It is not uncommon for press releases to be published in the news media exactly as they are written by university communication professionals, without any additional work or contextualization (Autzen 2014)—that is, the text read by the public is often the press release written by university communication professionals (Hansson 2017).

The aim of this chapter is thus to discuss how medical knowledge is adapted in the making of press releases, inspired by a particular field in the discipline of information studies concerned with what information artefacts such as books, articles, records, and other kinds of media do when they are embedded in sociocultural contexts and activities, and what people do with such information artefacts (Buckland 2012). Press releases can be seen as one kind of information artefact, which in addition to conveying a particular content also shapes activities and interaction between the parties involved in the writing and reading of these texts.

Method and material

The study is based on material gathered through semi-structured interviews with seven communication professionals and four neuroscience researchers working at medical faculties at two Swedish universities. The interviews lasted between 30 minutes and an hour. Some of the interviews were done by phone due to geographical distance between the author and the interviewee. The interviews concerned outreach activities and science communication in general. Press work and press releases were one theme included in the interview guide. Commonly, interviewees brought up this themselves before being asked about it. Press releases turned out to be something that all but one informant had some experience of or thoughts about. The press releases that were discussed by interviewees all reported medical scientific findings, and were written by communication professionals employed at medical departments or faculties at the two Swedish universities where the informants worked. These press releases have a characteristic form. The introductory sentences commonly state the name of the journal in which the reported findings have been published and the author's affiliation. They also include a link to the original journal article where the findings have been published, and the researchers' contact information. The findings and their implications are described briefly, and it is common to include quotes from interviews with the author of the journal article, and often a portrait image of the author, or, in cases when neuroscientific findings are reported, images of cells or brains.

The interviews were recorded, transcribed, and coded. The first round of coding identified the occurrence of broader, reoccurring, empirical themes. For this study, the press release theme was singled out and coded in further detail. Reoccurring themes identified were (*i*) how interviewees talked about findings in terms of breakthroughs; (*ii*) news; (*iii*) the importance of not promising too much; and (*iv*) the importance of encouraging the audience to identify with what is being reported. These themes will structure the empirical part of this chapter, exemplified by quotes from eight of the interviewees, duly anonymized—four communication professionals (Anna, Mary, Tom, and Sara) and four neuroscience scholars (Linda, Peter, Patricia, and Ivan). It should be noted that the focus is the communication professionals' and researchers' thoughts about press releases and their experiences, and the chapter does not aspire to gauge the audience's thoughts about or understanding of the press releases.

Genres as social action

Genre theory offers a useful approach for teasing out the disparities and similarities between various kinds of texts and what they are intended to achieve. The notion of genre can be understood in different ways, as referring to literary genres or more broadly to communicative activities (Andersen 2008, 2015; Kjellberg 2009). The latter notion, which is how genre will be used here, encompasses an understanding of genres as social action. Medical knowledge is communicated in many different ways, such as peer-reviewed journal articles, popular science books, blog posts, newspaper articles, and many more. These genres may be intended for different audiences and have different aims. Thinking of genres as communicative activities sheds light on how genres, in addition to facilitating the writing of texts, also enable their interpretation, setting out the connection between acts of writing, reading, and interpretation and other activities (Andersen 2015; Miller 1984). The conventions of a particular genre are not only applied when texts are written, but also when texts are read and made sense of. Understanding a text is not merely a matter of understanding the words; understanding also requires readers to grasp the conditions and situation in which a particular text was created. Through a shared understanding of how a genre is used and interpreted communicative activities are achieved. Hence, this understanding of genre implies that it is not only a way of representing content, but also a facilitator of social action. Genre is connected to particular communicative activities in which both writers and readers take part (Andersen 2015, 4). Genre theory draws attention to how content is mediated and the situations in which it is mediated, in addition to the form of the content. Sara Kjellberg's genre theoretical framework (2009) differentiates between four aspects of genre: aim, form, content, and context. Although they occasionally overlap, they are useful when identifying differences between types of texts. *Aim* refers to the purpose of the communicative act, that is, the intended purpose of the communication. *Form* refers to the ways the text is structured in such a way as to achieve the senders' intentions and the way in which the aim is conveyed. *Content* refers to what the text is about. *Context* concerns whom the communicator engages with and where communication occurs (Kjellberg 2009). This also involves communication in the contexts where particular texts are made. How the aspects of genre are manifested may vary over time, changing relative to transformations of the practices in which it is used. In this chapter, the insights of genre theory will be used to illuminate the differences and similarities between the genre of press releases and other related genres such as scholarly articles and news reports, as well as notions of what kind of communicative activities press releases are associated with. The context in question is the university, since this is where the communication professionals and researchers interviewed work.

Peer-reviewed journal articles and popular science

Though press releases can report any number of things, the ones discussed here concern medical scientific findings. Scholarly publications and popular science figure in many forms of publication, but are genres that in different ways are connected and related to press releases. The main features and differences between them will be identified in the light of previous research.

Scholarly communication is an established research field in information studies which encompasses the study of the writing, distribution, use, and citation patterns of scholarly publications (Borgman 2007; Cronin 2005). Though this research area may include both the formal and informal communication of research, the emphasis has primarily been on the exchange of ideas between scholars, although science in a number of formats is increasingly available to larger audiences, partly due to digital technologies (Borgman 2007, 48–9). Insights from this field of research provide a useful baseline for the aim, form, content and context of peer-reviewed journal articles. Scholarly publications may have different forms depending on the researcher's field, and the importance of different kinds of publications and genres vary between disciplines (Cronin 2005). In medicine, the discipline in focus in this chapter, the peer-reviewed journal article is the most important of all publications. The language of these publications is technical, and the intended readers are other medical scholars in the same research field. Whatever they publish, it must have the correct critical apparatus that connects it with previous publications in the field (Latour 1987), and new findings must similarly be presented in a way that connects with the established knowledge in the discipline (Borgman 2007, 47). The context in which articles are written and read is primarily an academic one. Bernd Frohmann (2004) has suggested that peer-reviewed journal articles are not only carriers of epistemic content, they also stabilize scientific fields and practices.

Previous studies of popular science writing, science journalism, and press releases have highlighted how scientific findings in these styles of writing differ from the conventions of writing for peer-reviewed journals.[1] These studies offer plenty of insights into aspects of popular science genres, although they have not applied genre theory. Many describe the form and content of popular science writing as featuring a sensationalist language not used in scientific journals (Fahnestock 1998; Johnson & Littlefield 2011; Nelkin 1996; Sismondo 2010). Sensationalist language may for example entail the use of superlatives such as the fastest, newest, and biggest, which was a recurring feature of science journalism throughout the twentieth century (Nelkin 1996). It is distinctive of popular science that writers adapt their message or information in such a way that it relates to values already held by non-expert audiences (Fahnestock 1998). This encompasses the identification of aspects that make findings attractive to readers who are not specialists in the particular area by appealing to wonder and how the findings can be applied. Jeanne Fahnestock (1998) suggests that popular science writing is about foregrounding certain aspects of the findings, and not about replacing technical terminology with words that are easier to comprehend. One technique is to frame findings in terms of breakthroughs (Fahnestock 1998). Such studies centre specifically on the language used in popular science, on the text itself, and not on the practices or the people or professionals involved in the writing. Narratives about science for public channels are not only a matter of conveying the results of particular studies, however, because they connect to larger issues and contribute to a sense that research and science can offer solutions to societal problems (Felt & Fochler 2012). Although written for readers who are not experts in the subject area, public accounts of science not only have consequences for the public's expectations of researchers, they also have consequences for how younger generations of specialists think of their role as researchers and what they see as important (Felt & Fochler 2012). Ulrike Felt and Maximilian Fochler (2012) suggest that the various kinds of activities that constitute science communication should be understood to be about creating and maintaining good relations between society and science.

Press releases

I discuss the aim, form, content, and context of the press releases based on four recurring themes identified in excerpts from interviews with public relations officers and senior researchers in the area of neuroscience. The first and second concern how findings are described in terms of news and breakthroughs; the third, making findings appear interesting to non-experts without instilling too much hope among patient groups; and the fourth, the significance of facilitating the reader's identification with the contents of the press release. Although overlapping, these themes are useful when pinpointing how medical knowledge is transformed as it circulates between practices.

News

Medical press releases may be intentionally addressed to particular audiences such as the media for medical professionals or other groups in healthcare settings. Most, however, are intended for media with broader audiences, and it was common for communication professionals to talk about the content of press releases as news.

> Anna: Research is like ready-made news, we don't have to make up strange investigations like other organizations may do. We have real news. That is something we see as a strength, then [our job] is about relating science and giving journalists support in writing about our researchers and what our researchers do.

Whether scientific findings really are news, how science and news relate to each other, and the similarities of 'science news' to other kinds of news can be discussed. Nik Brown (2003, 15) has stressed that science reports in the media differ from the common run of news. For something to qualify as a news story, it must report something that is both recent and has not been heard of before. What is reported in scientific publications, though, must connect to what is already known in the academic field in question (15). Brown writes that 'It is in fact extremely rare for something completely new to find its way into *Nature* or *Science*. Scientific news is more usually old news' (15).

The contexts of science and news reporting differ from each other. Rather than being out there, happening or being found, science news is constructed as such by journalists (Ideland 2002). Yet science news differs from other kinds of news such as reports on political events or decisions, for while that kind of news has a limited time frame, science news does not (44). With news only being news for a limited period of time, the implication is that journalists must work fast (Ideland 2002). The work that public relations officers do on press releases matches the pace of science journalism: they work fast and try to introduce findings in a concise manner that appeals to the media or the public. The interviewees emphasize the importance of fitting the science they report to these outlines. One of the communication professionals described the work involved in the distribution of press releases in the following way:

> Mary: —and then we discuss, how do we distribute this? This is really interesting, we should try to get it into [one of the larger news programmes on Swedish Television], this has potential… then you call [the news programme], one of the reporters, and say that we have this research, is that something [of interest], and you explain in a simple and fast manner what it is about. Yes, we are [they say], and then I send them the documentation, and at the same time I send it out widely and publish it on [the university's] website so when people hear about it on the news… they can always access the source. Because it can become distorted along the way. Irrespective of which channel, if we distribute [the press release] widely or do it more narrowly we always make sure that it is published on [the university website] at the same time, a text we can vouch for.

One of the points of a press release and the work surrounding it is to communicate science to audiences outside academia. Mary, a public relations officer, also touches on possible misrepresentations when it is picked up as 'news' by television, radio, or other news media. The same findings may be shaped to suit a different genre in a news context where texts adjust to other conventions of form and content. Something 'very exciting' may be misinterpreted, becoming something the academic institution may not want to be associated with. To maintain the connection to the academic context, this particular university makes sure that the original text is readily accessible on its website at the same time as the research features in the news. It is important to communication professionals and researchers alike to reduce the risk of misrepresentation, yet the composition of press releases requires the findings to be framed in certain ways in order to attract media attention.

Breakthroughs

Previous studies of the popularization of science have discussed how findings are conceptualized in terms of breakthroughs, or the possibility of describing findings in terms of a breakthrough (for example, Fahnestock 1998; Nelkin 1996). Attention is recognized by many interviewees in this study as an important factor in the press release genre, and by researchers as a reason why some findings gain publicity and others do not. Linda, a researcher, accepts this about press releases, and thus adjusts her involvement in making press releases, shaping their form and content, in accordance with what she finds appropriate. Not every study qualifies for the label of breakthrough, but in the writing of a press release acquires it en route, as if an unavoidable element of the genre. She therefore chooses her moment to go public with care.

> Linda: Sometimes you see press releases [about a colleague's work], studies that are actually quite uninteresting, about minimal progress, but that are emphasized in press releases as super interesting, and then the media take that as a starting point and write about it while you yourself know that this isn't really a breakthrough. In the media everything is a breakthrough, but in reality research doesn't work like that; not all studies lead to breakthroughs.

She touches on the tension between the way research is done and how the news media operate. There is something to process that means that breakthroughs figure more prominently in the press releases than they do in the research. Although Linda does not necessarily agree with this way of handling research findings, she is aware it is a feature of press releases that will contribute to its impact in the media. She knows what sort of communicative activity is intended, and what adaptions to the findings it requires. When Tom, who is a communications professional, describes which publications and findings are selected for press releases, he explains that the scientific community's evaluation is one important aspect, but not the only one taken into consideration. He talks explicitly about the importance of the findings being a breakthrough as a 'news hook' to catch the interest of readers. Indeed, his description highlights how important it is to know how press releases are both written and read in order to achieve their intended communicative activity.

> Tom: …and then I also have to see that there is a news hook, that there is a hook as it's called, something to attach the message to. And most commonly, the easiest way, is something like a breakthrough that is as close to the clinic or to a new treatment or therapy as possible.

The way Tom talks about news hooks echoes the features of popular science identified by Fahnestock (1998): it is not merely a matter of describing the findings in a non-technical manner, but of identifying the points that will give the message the greatest appeal to the intended audience. That the findings are considered a significant contribution to the field is one thing, but it is not the same thing as a news hook. One way to catch people's attention can be to emphasize closeness to a clinical application. An important feature of press releases is that in addition to announcing findings in a way that make them easy to comprehend, they also seek to generate exposure for the university (see Hansson 2005). Being very short, press releases are not the place for elaborate explanations of the findings, and certainly not in the detail one would expect to find in a research report.

> Sara: You can always tweak a little, and you always tweak a bit when you do a news angle because the headline must raise interest otherwise nobody will read [the press release]. You can't give the title of a dissertation as a headline but there must be some limits, not least when it concerns medicine, health, people's health and how people feel, there is a boundary when you have tweaked too much.

Like the other communication professionals interviewed in this study, Sara is cautious not to raise unrealistic expectations in patients (see Alftberg in this volume). Yet the rewriting of medical scientific findings as a press release necessarily involves some manipulation, some shifts in focus compared to the original publication. The job of the press release is to reach out and be read by non-experts, meaning that the structure and content of the two genres are very different.

The writing of press releases is accordingly one of adapting established medical knowledge in an academic field to the conventions of news reporting. There are recognized limits on how much recasting is acceptable, as noted by several of the communication professionals who were interviewed. These boundaries are handled by balancing the appeal to readers with avoiding high expectations among readers and patient groups.

Striking a balance

Choosing words and metaphors is a delicate issue when it comes to writing about medical advances. If a press release exaggerates or uses sensationalist language it may carry over into any news reports (Sumner et al. 2014). Much of the content and form of the popular science genres identifiable in previous studies does coincide with that highlighted by interviewees in this study. Excessive claims about the consequences of findings can be particularly problematic when press releases concern medical research, as the result can be hyped expectations among patient organizations and relatives that may not be met (Brown 2003). Audiences can perceive the same press release in differing ways: researchers, press officers, and patients' relatives may have very different understandings of what constitutes hype in a press release that reports medical science (Samuel et al. 2017). The communication professionals in this study acknowledge that the way knowledge is represented in press releases differs from the way the same findings are presented in journal articles. However, they are not indifferent to what this may entail, and particularly how the findings they describe might be interpreted and understood by patients. Striking a balance between giving findings general appeal and not instilling expectations that are too high is important. Much neuroscientific research is experimental and difficult for non-experts to grasp. Tom says that such research requires him to find a good angle—a suitable metaphor when describing the findings. Commonly, this angle will be the research's closeness to some new clinical application, but 'it is also very much about not creating too much expectation among patients. That is a key issue, to strike a balance each time, and that's something that you learn to calibrate, to stick to the right side of that line' (Tom). Communication professional Mary admits that mistakes are made, and gives a few examples of a lack of balance when writing press releases.

> Mary: We have made occasional faux pas, you make mistakes sometimes when you promise too much […] we may create enormous expectations among a group that suffers from severe illnesses and we shouldn't do that. We try to work [on that] and that is an act of balance, on one side trying to write something that carries a news value, and on the other make it interesting, and you are supposed to do that on an A4-sized page and simultaneously not instil expectations that are not realistic.

Writing a press release includes weighing up possible news values—what the public might find interesting—against the risk of raising expectations among patients and relatives that cannot be met, and doing all that in a very limited space.

Linda was one of those who made the point that reaching out to audiences outside academia requires a way of talking about research that is nothing like the conventions of scholarly publications. Likewise, Peter, another researcher, is aware of this, but chafes at the fact that this feature of press releases precludes an accurate account of research practice and the production of medical knowledge:

Peter: If you were to search for Parkinson's disease on [the university's] website you would find that Parkinson's enigma has been solved like 50 times here…
Author: You mean it has been written in that way?
Peter: Exactly, [inaudible] that's because that's the only way to reach out with your research and make someone interested in it. No one cares that we've taken a small step in Parkinson's research that will eventually, like in 50 years, contribute to solving the Parkinson's puzzle.

According to Peter, striving for visibility may lead to public pronouncements in which levels of certainty and research outcomes no longer correspond with what has actually been achieved. If this is the case, the writing and distribution of press releases is not primarily about accounting for findings, but a means for the university and researchers to gain visibility (for example, Samuel et al. 2017). In the science setting the findings may be a step forward, an advance on what is already known, but this may not be sufficient to garner public interest. Public attention, according to Peter, requires the exaggeration of both the issue investigated and the resultant findings. For one researcher, Patricia, who works in a lab far from the clinic and its patients, it may take time for findings to result in actual treatments and applications, yet she has a great deal of contact with patients, particularly following press releases.

Patricia: We had a publication in 2014 and a press release was made based on it. People still write and call to find out if they can test a new treatment and to find out what we are going to do now. I try to answer everything but sometimes I forget. In the beginning, I found this to be difficult. I thought, what are we supposed to say now? What if they interpret this in the wrong way? What if their expectations are exaggerated? Now I'm completely calm in this role, no severe consequences have resulted from my statements.

Patricia's reflections suggest that some experience is required in order to fully comprehend and handle the different communicative activities that the various genres generate. The literature describes press releases as partly responsible for raising unrealistic expectations among patients (for example, Brown 2003). That aspect to press releases does appear to be something that both communication professionals and researchers do their best to avoid, because they know what consequences it may have for patients. However, it might be impossible to completely avoid raising patients' hopes when doing research on human diseases (see Alftberg in this volume). That might not even be desirable. For patients and their relatives, hope may be a way of imagining a future (Nilsson & Hansson 2016). The quote from the interview with Patricia illustrates how press releases can also trigger or facilitate a dialogue between researchers and patients.

Identification

Which findings researchers may find interesting and which appeal to the news media and the public may differ. Responses from media may be wholly absent—or overwhelming. One of the interviewees, Ivan, expected as a researcher that a press release about a study he was involved in about the onset of Huntington's disease would gain far more public attention than it did.

> Ivan: …[we thought that] this will be really exciting, we could say that now we know why the onset of Huntington's disease occurs early or late [in a patient's life]. No, [a Swedish medical journal] wrote about it, that was that. Nobody else was interested, and then we thought is this too complicated? Is it too nerdy? Is Huntington's disease too unusual? Had it been Alzheimer's, would we have received more attention?

While the research group on this occasion considered their findings to be a major breakthrough, a considerable advance on what was known about Huntington's disease, the interest from the media was very low. Ivan wonders if the lack of interest is explained by Huntington's disease being rare; had their findings concerned the onset of a more common disease the response might have been different. Although by his account their findings did have what can be described as the makings of a breakthrough, the findings lacked relevance for a larger public. Being a breakthrough may thus not be sufficient for a finding to make a successful news story. Identification is an important feature in both science journalism and marketing, which may be achieved by evoking culturally established values. Popularized accounts or potentially controversial research seek to gain the approval of both the public and research funders (for example, Hansson 2005, 2006). Identification also appears to be central to the press release genre in terms of content. When reasoning about which press releases attract the media and public attention and which do not, the factor mentioned by both public relations officers and researchers was the bearing the findings in question had on something familiar to the public. The researchers' understanding of what deserves public attention does not necessarily coincide with what the general public can relate to or identify with. In Ivan's example, Huntington's disease may have been too rare for the press release to attract any wider publicity outside the medical professional community. On other occasions the media and public response can come as a surprise. Peter did not think the findings announced in his most recent press release to be particularly important, far less of any interest to audiences beyond the research community.

> Author: What happened the last time you did a press release?
> Peter: Well, the last time we did one it gained lots of visibility […]
> it was an experimental study, but the public relations officer put
> a very catchy title on the press release and that led to it gaining
> attention in the US. It was not widely distributed in Sweden, no
> news agencies or anything wrote about it. But in the US it was
> widely distributed.

The title chosen by the communication professional hinted that the findings could potentially make people smarter. Peter ascribes the attention the press release received not to the actual findings it reported, which according to him were minor, but to the catchy title chosen by the press officer that struck a chord with the public.

In addition to inherent newsworthiness, the intended readers' ability to relate to the message of the press release appears crucial to its ability to attract public interest. In other words, rather than announce something as completely new, an effective press release will make the findings sufficiently recognizable to fit with what is already familiar to the expected audience. In the genre of medical press releases, the content element is not merely a matter of accounting for breakthroughs or 'newish' findings in order for communication to be successful.

Conclusions

Although there may not be any firm boundaries between the scientific community and the public, there are differences in the genres used when communicating findings among researchers and audiences who are not medical experts. Genres differ in form and content, they do not have the same aims, and they are intended for a variety of contexts (Kjellberg 2009). The examples and material discussed here illustrate how medical knowledge adapts as it circulates between research practices and the practice of writing press releases. The differences between the genres used in these contexts demand adaption.

The communication professionals and researchers interviewed in this study generally have a shared understanding of the kind of communicative activities that press releases are intended to achieve when reaching out to non-academic audiences via the media. They also have a shared understanding of how research must be shaped in style and content in order for this to happen. In the interview material discussed above, press releases are described as connecting audiences and researchers based on scientific findings, the conventions of news reporting, and things familiar to non-experts.

Thinking in terms of genre as a communicative activity, the themes and examples considered here illustrate how press releases differ from academic publications in form. Press releases are clearly associated with visibility, accounting for something supposedly new yet familiar enough to make non-experts interested. The success of a press release does not depend on the importance ascribed to the findings by the research community, but on how well the reported findings could be represented in a way that corresponded with something the intended audience could relate to. One way of describing the work of writing press releases is that it is about taking findings designed to slot into the existing knowledge in an academic field and adapting them to the conventions of news reporting in terms of both content and form, reflecting their move into a different context, from scholarly publication into the news media.

Turning medical knowledge into press releases is not unproblematic. Points of tension are evident in the interviewees' reflections on the necessary negotiations when presenting findings in press releases, whether between research practice and how the news media works, and what each demands in order to be successful, or between an eagerness for visibility and a fear of building exaggerated expectations. When a balance is struck, however, a press release may not only operate as a mediator of visibility, but can also facilitate dialogue between researchers and patients. Scientific press releases constitute one kind of document that reports on popular science, retaining their ties to the scientific process by their connection to the original peer-reviewed publication of the findings, but also to the lives of non-scientists by accommodating the content, context, form, and aim in ways that non-experts can identify with.

Notes

1 This theme has been discussed by researchers from a variety of disciplines, for example STS (for example, Brown 2003; Felt & Fochler 2012), ethnology (for example, Hansson 2005; Ideland 2002), rhetoric (for example, Fahnestock 1998), literature (for example, Johnson & Littlefield 2012), and others (for example, Nelkin 1996; Sumner et al. 2014)

References

Aamodt, Sandra & Samuel Wang (2008), *Welcome to your brain: Why you lose your car keys but never forget how to drive and other puzzles of everyday life* (New York: Bloomsbury).

Andersen, Jack (2008), 'The concept of genre in information studies', *Annual Review of Information Science & Technology*, 42(1), 339–67.

—— (2015), 'What genre theory does', in id. (ed.), *Genre theory in information studies* (Bingley: Emerald).

Autzen, Charlotte (2014), 'Press releases—The new trend in science communication', *Journal of Science Communication*, 13(3), C02.

Borgman, Christine L. (2007), *Scholarship in the digital age: Information, infrastructure, and the Internet* (Cambridge, MA: MIT).

Brown, Nik (2003), 'Hope against hype—Accountability in biopasts, presents and futures', *Science Studies*, 16(2), 3–21.

Buckland, Michael K. (2012), 'What kind of science can information science be', *Journal of the American Society for Information Science & Technology*, 63(1), 1–7.

Cronin, Blaise (2005), *The hand of science: Academic writing and its rewards* (Lanham, MD: Scarecrow).

Damasio, Antonio R. (1994), *Descartes' error: Emotion, reason and the human brain* (London: Picador).

Fahnestock, Jeanne (1998), 'Accomodation science: The rhetorical life of scientific facts', *Written communication*, 15(3), 330–50.

Felt, Ulrike & Maximilian Fochler (2012), 'What science stories do: Rethinking the multiple consequences of intensified science communication', Department of Social Studies of Science, University of Vienna, December. http://sciencestudies.univie.ac.at/publications

Frohmann, Bernd P. (2004), *Deflating information: From science studies to documentation* (Toronto: University of Toronto Press).

Hansson, Kristofer (2005), 'Biopop: Biovetenskapens popularisering i medierna', *ETN: Etnologisk skriftserie*, 1(1), 107–117.

—— (2006), 'Den aktiva familjen i hälso- och sjukvården', in id. (ed.), *Etiska utmaningar i hälso- och sjukvården* (Lund: Studentlitteratur).

—— (2017), 'Mixed emotions in the laboratory: When scientific knowledge confronts everyday knowledge', in Kristofer Hansson & Marcus Idvall (eds.), *Interpreting the brain in society* (Lund: Arkiv).

Ideland, Malin (2002), *Dagens gennyheter: Hur massmedia berättar om genetik och genteknik* (Lund: Nordic Academic Press).

Johnson, Jenelle M. & Melissa M. Littlefield (2011), 'Lost and found in translation: Popular neuroscience in the emerging neuordisciplines', in Martyn Pickergill & Ira Van Keulen (eds.), *Sociological reflections on the neurosciences* (Bingley: Emerald).

Kjellberg, Sara (2009), 'Scholarly blogging practice as situated genre: An analytical framework based on genre theory', *Information Research*, 14(3).

Latour, Bruno (1987), *Science in action: How to follow scientists and engineers through society* (Cambridge, MA: Harvard University Press).

Miller, Carolyn R. (1984), 'Genre as social action', *Quarterly Journal of Speech*, 70(2), 151–67.

Nelkin, Dorothy (1996), 'An uneasy relationship: The tensions between medicine and the media', *The Lancet*, 347(9015), 1600–1603.

Nilsson, Gabriella & Kristofer Hansson (2016), 'Berättade fantasier om förr, nu och framtiden i vården av barn med diabetes', *Socialmedicinsk tidskrift*, 93(3), 261–70.

Samuel, Gabriell, Clare Williams & John Gardner (2017), 'UK science press officers, professional vision and the generation of expectations', *Public Understanding of Science*, 26(1), 55–69.

Seth, Anil & Chris Frith (2014), *30-second brain* (Sydney: Pier9).

Sismondo, Sergio (2010), *An introduction to science and technology studies* (Chichester: Wiley-Blackwell).

Sumner, Petroc, Solveiga Vivian-Griffiths, Jacky Boivin, Andy Williams, Christos A. Venetis, Aimée Davies, Jack Ogden, Leanne Whelan, Bethan Hughes, Bethan Dalton, Fred Boy & Christopher D. Chambers (2014), 'The association between exaggeration in health related science news and academic press releases: retrospective observational study', *BMJ*, 349:g7015.

PART III

CO-CREATION OF MEDICAL KNOWLEDGE

CHAPTER 5

The ethical tool
of informed consent

How mutual trust is co-produced through entanglements and disentanglements of the body

Markus Idvall

> I [doctor's name] have explained the plan and the aim of the study to [patient's name].

> I [patient's name] have been verbally informed about the study described above, have received the attached written information, and have had the opportunity to discuss its contents with the responsible doctor. I agree to participate in the study and I feel that my participation is wholly voluntary. I can at any time and without explanation stop my participation without this having any effect on my future care.

These statements are taken from a copy of an informed consent form that was used in a clinical trial, which a few years ago explored cell transplantation as a possible treatment for patients with Parkinson's disease. I received an unused electronic copy of the document from one of the researchers I interviewed as an example of how his research team had enrolled research subjects in the trial. The informed consent form was several pages long, its primary goal being to make individual patients consider whether to accept the possibility of undergoing a neurosurgical operation. Besides information about the different steps of the cell transplant research, the document comprised detailed information about risks and discomfort associated with the various tests and interventions. An MRI test, it was explained, can be experienced as strenuous because the subject has to be held still in a space which is confined and noisy. Implantation in the brain entails several risks, such as the spread of contaminants, but the surgery itself is associated with a risk for cerebral haemorrhage. Positive effects were also mentioned in the information sheet. Some patients who had undergone similar surgery earlier had been able to cut down on their anti-Parkinson's medication after the implantation. The paragraphs quoted above came on the last page of the consent sheet, and served as a transition into the part of the form where the doctor (the researcher) and the patient (the research subject) were to sign. The passage spelt out what the two sides were agreeing to: the doctor/researcher stated that they had 'explained the plan and the aim of the study', while the patient/research subject declared that they had been 'verbally informed about the study', had 'received the attached written information', and had had 'the opportunity to discuss' it.

Obviously, this was some kind of pledge that the two partners verbalized relative to each other. But what else is at stake in these few lines? What does it mean to give or obtain consent to participation in a research project in this way? What role does information or knowledge play in this context? In this chapter I will problematize how informed consent is practised in the everyday situations of a biomedical research process. In the analysis the focus will not be on the national legislation per se that exists as a foundation for how research subjects are informed about research participation, but rather the co-productive practices that constitute the informed consent procedures between research subjects and researchers. Informed consent, in a cultural analysis, is not only a signed document with legal connotations, but primarily an ethical tool for realizing research, and, as a consequence, a social process whereby the actors face each other under different circumstances. I will thus explore the constitution of the social process of informed consent, which researchers and research subjects and their respective allies—research nurses and family members—are engaged in, and thus learn more about informed consent as a co-production of mutual engagement and responsibility in the participating networks of the two negotiating sides.

Co-production and embodied entanglements

Informed consent, in its physical and non-physical forms, will thus be seen as a form of ethical tool that the two sides apply in relation to each other while simultaneously realizing clinical science. Informed consent is here closely linked to 'co-production', which is Sheila Jasanoff's term for how science, technology, and society operate together in the production of knowledge. In *States of Knowledge*, Jasanoff and colleagues (2004) enlarge on this perspective in a number of different kinds of contexts: climate science, science policy, genetic science, and so on. Central for my own work is Vololona Rabeharisoa and Michel Callon's chapter, 'Patients and scientists in French muscular dystrophy research', which develops an understanding of how lay interventions into biomedical research change the conditions for how scientists work. Rabeharisoa and Callon, who look at a patients' association's role in relation to science, focus on various aspects of a lay model of support for research. One of these aspects concerns 'the tools' applied by the patients' association for 'the orientation, the steering and the evaluation' of how it supports research (Rabeharisoa & Callon 2004, 144). My focus will be on how informed consent—just like the films, photographs, books, and testimonies in Rabeharisoa and Callon's examples—operates as a tool for the orientation, steering, and evaluation for how scientists and patients collaborate in order to make clinical research ethical and thus feasible.

Thus I draw on both Jasanoff's and Rabeharisoa and Callon's discussions of co-production to distinguish that the knowledge that was co-produced in the cell transplant research information procedures was not the type of new biomedical knowledge that eventually changes people's treatments, or even their ways of being cured. Rather, what was co-produced in this process was a sort of shared information about the other side, which in the long run may in part be beneficial for how the other type of knowledge, the findings, may be achieved, but which in the process of the trial was essentially about establishing co-productive trust between the two sides. Informed trust, rather than consent, is in this way co-produced through what Rabeharisoa and Callon call 'mutual learning' (2004, 144) (see also Hansson & Irwin in this volume). Scientists learn about the participants by securing individual patients for the research project, and simultaneously listening to the questions and concerns that these participants have. The participants in their turn learn about the research by seeking answers to their own questions in the information process and by listening strategically to the scientists. Therefore, unlike Rabeharisoa and Callon, I focus on individuals in action rather than on a model of an organization. On the pathway of the informed consent procedure, along which information circulates between the two sides and also transforms the positions of the two sides into networks of participating actors, a platform for new biomedical knowledge (and technologies) is co-produced.

In the midst of this co-production is a form of mutual, ethical labour based on the specific tool of informed consent, which centres on the human body in that particular situation, and where the objective is not only to entangle the body in the action, but also to disentangle it from the context that eventually may appear. In *Tissue Economies*, Catherine Waldby and Robert Mitchell (2006, 60) write of one type of economic entanglement and disentanglement as 'analytical categories … to explore how embryos move from the human body to clinics, laboratory, and stem cell banks'. A stem cell bank, according to Waldby and Mitchell, 'performs a complex double role' when it manages its 'complex regimes of ontological, ethical, therapeutic, and commercial value' (60).

> On the one hand, it [the stem cell bank] assists in the technical work of disentangling tissues by facilitating the donation, stand-

ardization, and global circulation of stem cells. Yet on the other hand, it performs ethical work that involves a certain re-entanglement, for by placing certain limits on the marketing of cell lines and the commercialization of research, it attempts to divert the epistemological value of research into the categories of the public good and the national health. (Waldby & Mitchell 2006, 60)

In the case of the informed consent procedure studied here, the process of how the human body is made useful to research goes from entanglements of the human body to disentanglements—something which will be clarified below in a discussion of the move from teaching consent to de/signing (of which more later), documenting and, finally, reporting consent.

Material and method

Before I turn to the question of informed consent, I want to say a few words about fieldwork. Parkinson's disease, the disorder on which I concentrated in my fieldwork, is a neurodegenerative disease that was first designated by the British doctor James Parkinson (1755–1824) in the early nineteenth century. The cause of the disease, however, is still unknown. The disease is elicited by the continuous death of a certain type of cell in the brain: dopamine cells. With the loss of these cells specific symptoms arise: rigidity, shaking, problems with balance, and loss of the power of voluntary movement. Non-motor symptoms such as tiredness, sleeping problems, anxiety, depression, and dementia can also develop. Different pharmaceutical treatments, including levodopa, have an effect on the symptoms, but cannot cure the disease itself. Moreover, these treatments function well only in the beginning; ultimately the positive effects are reduced and instead side effects develop, for example dyskinesias (impairment of voluntary movements) (Hagell 2004, 78 ff.). Parkinsonism is therefore the target of many clinical trials in the world today. The scientists use different kinds of approaches in order to understand the disease better and to find new treatments for the condition. The research focus shifts between neuroprotective strategies, the role of physical exercise, genetic disposition, cell transplantations, and so on (Palfreman 2015). For some years (2012–18) I had the opportunity to learn more about this research when I conducted fieldwork at a university clinic that specializes in research on Parkinson's disease. I happened to focus on cell transplantation research, but I also encountered other types of biomedical research, for example the mapping of genetic heritage and the implantation of human growth factor. My fieldwork was conducted at intervals and included various methods: observations, focus-group interviews, individual interviews, etc. (Idvall et al. 2013; Idvall 2017a–b). Here I will examine the individual interviews and how this part of the fieldwork, conducted between 2015 and 2018, revealed a form of split collaboration between researchers and research subjects regarding how the two relate to clinical trials and informed consent.

The interviewed researchers were a relatively homogeneous professional staff of five doctors and five research nurses. Two out of the five doctors specialized in cell transplantations. The research subjects who I interviewed were a more heterogeneous category, with individuals with Parkinson's disease as well as relatives of some of those affected. Nine individuals with Parkinson's disease were interviewed individually, while seven individuals were interviewed together with a family member. Only three individuals had first-hand experience of cell transplantation research; however, several individuals had experience of taking part in medical research, and those few who did not were able to talk about science and clinical trials from a perspective that included their personal experience of living with the illness.

In the individual interviews I took an ethnographic approach to learn more about the cultural encounters between researchers and research subjects (Idvall 2005). I tried to map how the co-production of informed consent was realized between researchers and research subjects. Doctors and research nurses were asked how they went about obtaining informed consent from potential participants in the clinical trials, and we discussed how they as scientific staff retained consent during the trials and what role consent played afterwards. In interviewing the research subjects, I likewise charted their experiences of the process of informed consent in a clinical trial. Individuals with Parkinson's disease and, where relevant, their family members were asked how they had consented, their experiences of taking part in a research project, their understanding of the information given by the medical staff, and the extent to which they felt themselves to be autonomous in their decisions. Those interviewees who did not have personal experience of taking part in a clinical trial discussed the topic on the basis of their illness experience.

Teaching consent

In the event, my analysis of co-productive practices as the realization of mutual consent was sparked by an observation rather than an interview. That moment came at the beginning of my fieldwork. I was in an audience of around 40 in a lecture room on the very top floor of a university hospital building, the panoramic view of the city darkening as the sun went down. We in the audience were mostly strangers to one another, but I suspected many had Parkinson's disease or were family members, since they all were of the age when Parkinson's disease usually first presents, that is in their fifties, sixties, or seventies. A few had visible symptoms of the disease, however, and then there was a scattering of my own sort—medical and social scientists.

The critical moment of the evening, which I remember so clearly, was when the first speaker, a senior specialist, started his presentation. Everyone listened carefully because he was well known as a successful, experienced clinical scientist at the university clinic. He had been part of the clinical trials conducted in the 1980s, and he was expected to be involved in new clinical trials in the near future. In his presentation, he gave an overview of the status of the ongoing research and listed some of the challenges ahead.

I experienced his presentation as professional and objective. He gave no unfounded promises; his was a realistic account of what the immediate future might hold. The audience seemed satisfied with his picture of things. Still, they had a great many questions afterwards. One of course was when clinical trials were expected to start. The specialist, whose calm and neutral way of reasoning never deserted him, could not point to any specific time.

He was not the only speaker that evening. Two people with Parkinson's disease also gave presentations. Like the specialist, they were quite well known to the audience, being leading patient activists. On this occasion they presented their views on what science can do for patients with Parkinson's disease and their families. What struck me was that their presentations gave us a more personal view on how scientists and patients can work together to achieve new treatments for Parkinson's disease. Both had a grasp of the science and could discuss their disease using scientific insights—but they could also talk about their personal experience of the disease in a compellingly authentic way. The audience seemed enthusiastic. Like the senior specialist, the two patients were peppered with questions and reflections afterwards.

During my time with the biomedical research programme I attended three or four co-productive events of this sort. What I encountered at these events were two kinds of objective, embodied ways of relating to the biomedical knowledge that was discussed. On the one hand, there were the explanations by the scientists, who spoke and 'framed' the issues individually and mostly from the front of the lecture room. They were, in Anthony Giddens's words (1991, 109–143), the expertise at these events. On the other hand, I saw a different kind of participation, which was more indirect and personal and mostly realized in the seats of the lecture room—what laypeople do when following discussions about scientific progress on-site. In this case it was, in Giddens's perspective, more a manifestation of lay views on biomedical knowledge, which hold a great deal of embodied expertise in the specific setting.

These events, flagged as science cafés, were arranged on the initiative of members of a highly prestigious research programme on cell transplantation that hoped to launch new clinical trials with Parkinson's patients within a few years. Inspired by the French tradition of *cafés scientifiques* (Russell 2010, 92–3), they were meant as a way of communicating science in mutual dialogue with people in general and patients in particular. The plan was to have at least two meetings a year, one in the spring and one in the autumn. Mainly it was seen as a possibility for patients and relatives to learn about the science that was taking place at the university hospital, but it was also for the scientists to learn about the families and their situation. The unspoken ambition was that laypeople and scientists would meet as equals at these events (Russell 2010, 92–3).

What the science cafés represent is a keen co-productive approach, which it was hoped would overflow into how scientists and participants work together in clinical trials. With their lectures and audiences, they may be seen as a form of start-up for the patients' participation in clinical trials; an active learning platform where potential subjects in future trials and their family members can find out about the science involved. Listening to a specialist give a lecture is like reading the patient association's periodical (*Parkinsonjournalen*)—a way to take responsibility and be informed about one's own illness. A central aspect of this learning moment is that all the individuals are exposed to the instrumental use of Parkinsonism bodies in clinical science, and are forced to imagine their own body's possible 'usefulness' in upcoming trials (see Goodman et al. 2003).

For the clinical scientists, in their turn, it is important that patients reflect on the research. The more conscious their patients are about the science, the easier it is for the scientists to do science—that at least appears to be the argument. Transparency turns out to be a crucial ideal for scientists and research nurses. But of course, theirs is a partial or tactical transparency. There is no question of full openness about what takes place in laboratories and operation theatres; rather, a relative openness that can interest people in supporting developments (Idvall 2003). As patient, one becomes entangled in the scientific process and feels more and more committed to the goals that science offers in that particular situation.

De/signing consent

The process of informed consent can start in the lecture room or the science café, but the document itself—the co-productive tool—is never in evidence at this stage. As a patient, one can add one's name to a list to receive further information about the research, or, like one research subject did, hand one's business card to a lecturing researcher, but the informed consent form will not be produced until the moment comes to enrol potential participants in a clinical trial. This is done by the researchers who plan and design the project's procedure of informed consent. The informed consent form is drawn up in a pre-phase of the clinical trial. In drafting the research protocol, the scientists turn to an ethics committee and propose a procedure for how to recruit patients to the project with informed consent: the principal investigator is thus responsible for the design of the informed consent procedure in dialogue with the ethics committee. The protocol, which directs everything in the research project, is central to how informed consent is structured and put into practice.

Subjects are not presented with an informed consent form until they are to be enrolled in a trial. The co-productive tool is part of a process that often begins with the clinical scientists approaching patients who they have met in the clinic—their 'own' patients— although in some cases others who do not attend the clinic contact the scientists and ask to take part in a study (see Hansson 2017). One clinical scientist (Interview no. 19) explained that when this happens she needs to judge whether the person is eligible to be a research participant. For example, she has to consider whether there are indications of 'cognitive weakness', or a tendency to fail to come to appointments. As a scientist she never says yes immediately, for example by email. Instead, she asks the patients to send her copies of their medical notes (*patientjournal*). Sometimes she has to reject patient requests when they do not meet the study's inclusion criteria.

The informed consent form is signed either at the potential research subject's home or at the university clinic; where exactly will depend on the nature of the research project—whether it is invasive or not—and whom the patients are to interact with. When the research project in question is less invasive it is expected that potential participants can make the decision on their own or together with a family member, in which case they usually sign at home. They may receive a letter from the clinic, asking that if they agree they return the completed consent form back to the clinic. In more invasive studies, potential participants may receive information at home, but wait until their next meeting at the clinic to sign there in the company of a doctor or a nurse.

With a co-productive approach, in the early phase of recruiting research subjects and possibly obtaining consent, both written and verbal information is included. Some of the interviewees stated that the written information was the most important for them. One man (Interview no. 6) who took part in a trial together with his wife felt that he needed to revisit the information more than once. This is an important argument for having written information: to be able to reread it at home, with extra time to consider one's options. It can also be a way to discuss the alternatives with one's family. One interviewee (Interview no. 12) thought that verbal information can always be misunderstood, and he needed written information in order to be able to discuss it with his wife at home, whom he felt was more perceptive than he was about this kind of question.

However, verbal information had its proponents too. One woman (Interview no. 5) explained that the verbal information made it possible for her to put direct questions about the surgery to the clinical scientist. Another interviewee (Interview no. 15) described how he accepted participation in a trial on the spot. He was not interested in reading any information, the verbal information had convinced him to participate because some of the scientists who were responsible for the project had been involved in earlier trials, and therefore in his view had important insights about how best to do this new project. This research subject was focused on the scientists' authority rather than on the risk–benefit assessment offered in the written information.

Proof, verification or contract?

What does the signed consent form, the two signatures, represent for the individuals concerned? For the researchers, the two signatures are proof that information has been given and consent has been obtained in that specific situation. Regarding signing, the scientists explained that by doing so they certified that the research subject had had the chance to ask them questions. One research nurse (Interview no. 21) stressed that the act of signing is an active stance by the participants. The signed consent form here becomes a kind of declaration of responsibility which the participants express towards science. Signing, in the eyes of the scientists, also becomes a way of preventing patients from taking participation too lightly: some are 'quite fast' when deciding to take part in a study. As a clinical scientist, one needs to make sure that the patients really have read the information and understood it. A patient must from this viewpoint be aware that by signing a consent form they have a responsibility to understand the information that they have received.

Proof was perhaps not what the research subjects first thought of when they reflected on the meaning of informed consent. Still, a few realized that the signing of the consent form was more for the scientists than for the sake of the subjects. One woman and her husband (Interview no. 8) said that by signing it protects the scientists; it gives them carte blanche in that particular situation. The signing of the consent form means that the scientists are taking a belt and braces approach—'både hängslen och livrem'—in order to be certain in their work, as one participant put it (Interview no. 3). However, most of the interviewees agreed on what the scientists thought about it—signing is a sort of verification of their responsible participation in clinical science. Perceptions of responsibility can in this way be something that all participants experience when signing a consent form. One woman (Interview no. 5) explained that she had a responsibility as a research subject; one should not withdraw from a research project on a whim, or mismanage one's medication, if participating in a trial. For another of the interviewees (Interview no. 9), consent in writing was 'a type of contract', since participation in the trial would be 'a big thing'.

In sum, the de/signing of the informed consent form appears to be, as Nikolas Rose (1999, 154) would have it, a form of governing style where 'responsibilization' becomes an essential cultural ingredient in how individuals act towards research within the frames of a neoliberal society. Responsibilization here is intimately linked with a certain degree of parallel freedom—'autonomization', as Rose calls it—for both the research subjects and the scientists: a dyadic or co-productive process of governing, which, as will be seen, is essential in the next phase of how informed trust is formed.

Documenting consent

In the phase of the research process when the participants are subject to different tests and interventions, signed consent becomes a tool that exists both on paper and as an electronic copy in a range of contexts. The participant's signed consent form is saved in the original in a folder that is stored in a locker or on a shelf in a locked room. The signature therefore exists as a physical object, safely archived in the university hospital for the lifetime of the research project. Electronically, the signed consent form is also included in the participant's medical notes, making their participation in the clinical trial plain to all their caregivers.

A paper copy of the signed consent form is also offered to the participants themselves. In this case the signed form exists as a reminder of an action in the past, brought home for keeping by a multitude of individuals with different routines for saving medical information and 'important papers'.

This anxious documenting of informed consent reflects the fact that consent is always negotiable, and in that sense must be defended throughout a research process. The fragility of mutual trust stems from the continuous straddling of the co-production process between Rose's two principles of responsibilization and autonomization (1999). The signed informed consent form is, as we have seen, a responsibilization tool, but it only works as long as both sides—the researchers and the patients—know they can act with autonomy relative to the other. For the researchers, this autonomy comes with the act of documenting consent. Armed with this documentation, the researchers have some sort of recourse when faced by unexpected events not of their own making. In some instances, research subjects can misunderstand or even forget what they have consented to. For the doctors and nurses, the archived consent form can serve as proof in dealings with research subjects who fail to comprehend what they approved to earlier. The document is almost never referred to in this process. However, if a patient were to forget a test or intervention needed in order to fulfil the project criteria, the research staff can discharge their responsibility by showing the patient the document, even though, given the situation, they might not insist on continuing the collaboration.

Thus, if discharge is a way out for the researcher, withdrawal is what the research subjects can do in order to assert their autonomy in relation to the research project. The withdrawal alternative is included in the informed consent agreement from the beginning. If a research subject decides to withdraw they do not have to explain why; it is a way out that does not have to be defended. In my interviews with research participants, none had withdrawn, even though some had been disappointed by their participation in a project. One man (Interview no. 15) told me that he started in an observation group before he was randomized into a transplant group, but after a while he was resassigned to the control group of the cell transplant study. This was very hard on him psychologically. He had got used to the idea that he was going to have a transplant, and nursed the hope that he would be cured. He indicated his disappointment with his participation in the biomedical research throughout the interview. Still, when I asked him if he was considering withdrawing from the project he replied without hesitation that he was not.

As previous studies show (Brown 2003; Lundin 2004; Novas 2006; Rubin 2008), patients have expectations of their participation in research projects. A certain treatment can be a reason for participation, with the project a chance to get something beyond the regular treatments. One of my interviewees (Interview no. 10) spoke frankly of considering withdrawing from a project when he realized that he was not going to get the experimental treatment he was hoping for. Finding himself in the control group, he sensed that he no longer had a goal. It felt like 'a kick in the stomach' when he realized he was not going to get the cells and, as he saw it, eventually be cured. Still, he decided to stay in the project, and afterwards he felt he could use his experience against the project—for example, when he attended a hospital appointment abroad in order to take some tests which were mandatory for the trial, he ordered, at the expense of the research project, a hotel room that was a bit larger than standard and he also got a special flight ticket. Moreover, when the scientists heard that he was considering opting out, it was his impression that they offered him something in return if he stayed on: after the project was finished, he would be going to be first in line for participation in two other projects that were about to start. In effect they offered him, as the participant expressed it, 'a small sack of candy'. The promise of being prioritized as a candidate for other studies with experimental treatments can be motivation enough for people in the control group of a clinical trial.

The motives for withdrawing have many elements. Disappointment is one of them. Being a research subject is in itself a vulnerable position and, like Tove Godskesen (2015) demonstrates in her dissertation *Patients in Clinical Cancer Trials*, may in some instances generate unrealistic hopes among individuals, which can eventually lead to great disappointment as well. However, it does not always have to be disappointment that drives someone to withdraw from a project. In my material, it happens mostly because research subjects become more ill or experience growing tiredness due to their chronic disorder. One way of handling this kind of risk of withdrawal is for the research staff to offer participants house calls instead of meeting them at the hospital. A scientist together with a research nurse may decide to conduct the tests on the trial participants at home, sparing participants the journey to the hospital.

Withdrawal and discharge are thus essential aspects of auto-nomization for how the documentation phase of the trial process eventually moves on to the stage when the results are ready to be communicated in various scientific contexts. In this latter phase, which ostensibly ends the participation of the trial subjects, mutual trust between researchers and participants is still defended in the form of the ethical format of the scientific periodicals.

Reporting consent

> The protocol was reviewed and approved by the institutional re-view board of each participating centre as well as the performance and safety monitoring board of the National Institutes of Health. After providing written informed consent, patients underwent laboratory screening and were excluded from further participation if they had evidence of infection with human immunodeficiency virus, hepatitis, or syphilis. (Olanow et al. 2003, 404)

The quote is from a scientific article in which a number of North American scientists described a cell transplant study where placebo surgery had been used to study the effect and survival of foetal cells in the brain of Parkinson's subjects. These surgeries were not uncontroversial, and gave rise to an ethical debate about whether it was acceptable to use placebo or sham surgery on the research subjects under such circumstances (Idvall 2017a, 132–6). In the article, the research subjects' written consent to participate in the research is treated as little more than a technicality—'After providing written informed consent' is all that is said about the presumably long process of teaching, de/signing, and documenting consent— and as such the consent process is reduced to an anonymous and collective event in the past. Each individual informed act of consent is not communicated. Instead, what is reported is a type of collective consent, summarizing how a whole group chose to become research participants.

After clinical trials have ended, informed consent thus loses its character as evidence for the scientists and instead becomes an active element in the reporting of the results. Usually the obligatory section on methods and source materials in a scientific article includes a description of how the informed consent procedure was conducted. It is rarely as brief as in the article quoted above, but regardless, what is said about the consent procedure is essential in the reporting context. Without this ethical format, biomedical scientists may not be allowed to publish their results in scientific periodicals, since most journals have rules which prohibit publication if informed consent is not reported in the study.

The anonymous reporting of collective consent may be seen as an example of a disentanglement of the particular embodied 'gift' which the 'useful body' of the research subject represents in the context of clinical studies. Waldby and Mitchell's discussion (2006, 69–73) of how embryos, as body parts used in science, emerge out of embodied social relations, but are disentangled from this complexity by means of informed consent processes, is eye-opening in this respect. They describe informed consent as a form of surrogate property contract between recipients and donors. Informed consent becomes a way for the recipient of embryonic cells and tissues to disentangle the embodied gift from the donor, as well as the complex context in which the donated cells and tissues have their origin, making it possible for the recipient to take control of the embodied gift.

In cell transplant research the disentanglement that reporting consent achieves means that researchers ultimately take symbolic control of the research subjects' bodies—those 'useful' bodies that were examined and subjected to interventions in the earlier stages of the research process, but which are now transformed into numbers and figures. For the research subjects themselves, the disembodying of individual consent that disentanglement leads to becomes a question of how to continue their participation in science. Taking part in a clinical trial is often associated with the chance of obtaining more information than patients in general. Participants seem to expect communications that are adjusted to their ability to understand the essentials of the results. In my interviews with research subjects, many felt they lacked information about how far the research was from a breakthrough or a new discovery. Perceptions of slowness of science were ubiquitous among patients and their family members. The time frame set by what they perceived as the slow progress of science (Idvall 2017b; see also Wiszmeg 2019) far exceeded their own lifetimes. One patient (Interview no. 11) explained that she had had Parkinson's disease for more than ten years. During that period she had heard about stem cells continuously, but nothing happens, she exclaimed. A man (Interview no. 14) who had been ill for twelve years thought that things did not move fast enough for the scientists. He felt that a lot more could be done, but he guessed that there was not enough funding.

The lack of information can be quite unsettling for many participants. One research subject (Interview no. 10) expressed his frustration at getting very little information, saying that no one asked how the 'rat' felt (his way of articulating his sense of being a guinea pig). He added that participants and scientists will never be equals, since the participant does not have a clue about what the scientist is doing and the scientist has a 'helicopter perspective'. Similarly, one woman (Interview no. 5) said that she felt a disadvantage next to the scientists, since she had not received any results or information after her last tests. Another person (Interview no. 11) explained that only a 'short call about the benefits' of the research that she had participated in would have been 'enough' to make it acceptable. One couple (Interview no. 14) acknowledged that their research participation felt a bit 'thin' after they received no feedback about the findings following the tests. A man (Interview no. 15) who was currently participating in a project complained that he had not had any information about research outcomes, whether personally from the researchers or from the project website, because of that he felt he had no influence at all on the research.

The opposite can also be the case, for not all participants are interested in the results. As one man (Interview no. 6) explained, it was a good thing that he and his wife joined in a clinical trial, but they were never really interested in the potential findings. Another interviewee (Interview no. 7) emphasized that one does not have to be interested in the specific research project in order to participate. It is more a question of being willing to help for the good of all—it is part of one's responsibility, as she said.

Movements of informed consent

I have shown how the co-production of biomedical knowledge and mutual trust are dependent on the ethical tool of informed consent, which involves a process of negotiation between scientists and participants. In this process, informed consent takes different forms—verbal, paper, electronic—and goes through different phases. In an early phase, scientific cafés can be a way of establishing an effective co-productive dialogue between researchers and research subjects. A teaching mode is central to preparing for informed consent. In the recruiting phase the actual negotiation starts between the scientists and the participants. A critical decision-making situation is struck up between individuals, representing the two negotiating parties when the consent form is designed and signed: a form of entangling responsibilization is enacted by researchers and research subjects in a mutual dialogue. Further on, in the test and intervention phase, the fragility of informed consent is a consequence of different techniques of autonomization. Withdrawal is open to research subjects who are too ill, tired, or disappointed to continue. For scientists, freedom is grasped through the sort of discharge of responsibility that a completed informed consent form can offer in situations of uncertainty and disagreement. In the final phase, informed consent procedures can be traced in the scientific publications, often in the sections on material and method. By this stage the individual bodies of the research subjects have been disentangled from the embodied social relations of the original informed consent. At the same time the research subjects can experience this end-phase of the scientific project as marking their exclusion from information flows and from actual participation.

Thus, teaching, de/signing, documenting, and reporting consent and mutual trust together make up the various aspects of an embodied ethics, which deals with the moral dilemmas of clinical science and the vitality of the human body (Rose 2007, 254), but which also, paradoxically, includes a disembodying factor, through the impact of the scientific journals, that blurs and de-personalizes how the knowledge was originally co-produced.

References

Brown, Nik (2003), 'Hope against hype: Accountability in biopasts, presents and futures', *Science Studies*, 16(2), 3–21.

Giddens, Anthony (1991), *Modernity and self-identity: Self and society in late modern age* (Cambridge: Polity).

Godskesen, Tove (2015), *Patients in clinical cancer trials: Understanding, motivation and hope* (Acta Universitatis Upsaliensis; Uppsala: Uppsala universitet).

Goodman, Jordan, Anthony McElligott & Lara Marks (2003) (eds.), *Useful bodies: Humans in the service of medical science in the twentieth century* (Baltimore: John Hopkins University Press).

Hagell, Peter (2004), 'Utmaningar i utvecklingen: Nya behandlingsmetoder av Parkinsons sjukdom', in Susanne Lundin (ed.), *En ny kropp: Essäer om medicinska visioner och personliga val* (Lund: Nordic Academic Press).

Hansson, Kristofer (2017), 'Mixed emotions in the laboratory: When scientific knowledge confronts everyday knowledge', in Kristofer Hansson & Markus Idvall (eds.), *Interpreting the brain in society: Cultural reflections on neuroscientific practices* (Lund: Arkiv).

Idvall, Markus (2003), 'Främmande kunskap: Informationens strategiska betydelse för utvecklingen av xenotransplantation', in Fredrik Schoug & Markus Idvall (eds.), *Kunskapssamhällets marknad* (Lund: Studentlitteratur).

—— (2005), 'Intervjun som kulturlaborativ praktik', paper at ACSIS Kulturstudier i Sverige: Första nationella forskarkonferensen, Norrköping 13–15 June, ISSN online 1650-3740.

—— Andréa Wiszmeg & Susanne Lundin (2013), *Focus group conversations on clinical possibilities and risks within Parkinson's disease: A Swedish case study* (Lund: Department of Arts and Cultural Sciences, Lund University).

—— (2017a), 'Taking part in clinical trials: The therapeutic ethos of patients and public towards experimental cell transplantations', in Kristofer Hansson & Markus Idvall (eds.), *Interpreting the brain in society: Cultural reflections on neuroscientific practices* (Lund: Arkiv).

—— (2017b), 'Synchronizing the self with science: How individuals with Parkinson's disease move along with clinical trials', *Ethnologia Scandinavica*, 47, 57–77.

Jasanoff, Sheila (2004) (ed.), *States of knowledge: The co-production of science and social order* (London: Routledge).

Lundin, Susanne (2004), 'Etik som praxis', in ead. (ed.), *En ny kropp: Essäer om medicinska visioner och personliga val* (Lund: Nordic Academic Press).

Novas, Carlos (2006), 'The political economy of hope: Patients' organizations, science and biovalue', *BioSocieties*, 1(3), 289–305.

Olanow, C. Warren, C. G. Goetz, J. H. Kordower, A. J. Stoessl, V. Sossi, M. F. Brin et al. (2003), 'A double-blind controlled trial of bilateral fetal nigral transplantation in Parkinson's disease', *American Neurological Association*, 54(3), 403–414.

Palfreman, John (2015), *Brain storms: The race to unlock the mysteries of Parkinson's disease* (New York: Scientific American/Farrar, Straus & Giroux).

Rabeharisoa, Vololona & Michel Callon (2004), 'Patients and scientists in French muscular dystrophy research', in Jasanoff 2004.

Rose, Nikolas (1999), *Powers of freedom: Reframing political thought* (Cambridge: CUP).

—— (2007), *The politics of life itself: Biomedicine, power, and subjectivity in the twenty-first century* (Princeton: PUP).

Rubin, Beatrix P. (2008), 'Therapeutic promise in the discourse of human embryonic stem cell research', *Science as Culture*, 17(1), 13–27.

Russell, Nicholas (2010), *Communicating science: Professional, popular, literary* (Cambridge: CUP).

Waldby, Catherine & Robert Mitchell (2006), *Tissue economies: Blood, organs, and cell lines in late capitalism* (Durham: Duke University Press).

Wiszmeg, Andréa (2019), *Cells in culture, cells in suspense: Practices of cultural production in foetal cell research* (Lund: Department of Arts and Cultural Sciences, Lund University).

CHAPTER 6

The co-creation of situated knowledge

Facilitating the implementation of care models in hospital-based home care

Kristofer Hansson, Gabriella Nilsson & Irén Tiberg

In recent decades, it has become standard for health care, both medical treatments and nursing praxis, to be based on research, so-called evidence-based care. Healthcare has increasingly come to operate on an evidence-based paradigm, with its rationale that research should have a stronger position. This applies not only to changes in treatment routines, but also to views on how patients and their relatives should be treated, and what constitutes the best, most appropriate care. The implementation of research-based knowledge in care praxis has proved difficult and cannot be said to happen by itself. It is therefore crucial to further develop existing implementation methods, in order to facilitate the application of research findings in practice by integrating them into existing care praxis (Barrett 2004; Saetren 2005; Richards & Rahm Hallberg 2015).[1]

Thus, the research-based knowledge to be implemented in a healthcare setting amounts to an ontology of sorts, which brings with it certain ways of considering such entities as healthcare, patients, treatment, and so on (Law 1996; Mol 1999, 2002). A consequence is, when research-based knowledge is to be put into daily practice—when the research model is to be translated into care practice—there is a risk that differences of opinion will arise if these findings are misunderstood, obstructed, or result in unintended practices; dissent then becomes apparent when implementing new care models, where research-based knowledge conflicts with the values behind the health professionals' existing practices, habits, and ideas (Nilsson et al. 2018).[2]

This chapter explores the potential of using ethnographic methods to support medical personnel who are in the process of replacing existing practice with a new research-based care practice—in other words, when an new evidence-based care model is operationalized (see also Woolgar 1988; Ashmore 1989; Bragesjö 2004). The method presented here centres on offering support to the member of the medical team who is to facilitate the actual implementation—the so-called facilitator—so the team can better understand the processes at work (Tiberg et al. 2017). The purpose is to highlight how ethnographic methods can make the facilitator's task of driving the implementation easier.

Research-based, evidence-based

Before describing the ethnographic method, the project and the importance of implementation in the healthcare sector will be discussed by addressing the growing interest in scientific evidence (see Irwin in this volume). Internationally, there has been a move towards evidence-based healthcare in recent decades (Bohlin & Sager 2011; Richards & Rahm Hallberg 2015). This is in part because evidence-based healthcare is thought to promote equitable, high-quality care by reducing variations in healthcare provision, which might otherwise leave some patients without access to the best available care. Another reason is that there is a gap between healthcare praxis and the research findings that are available, which leads to care that is less effective and, at worst, harmful to the patient (Svensk sjuksköterskeförening 2016). This is the case made by the WHO (2006), concerned by the challenges facing health services because of increasingly stretched resources.

The example presented here is an evidence-based care model

designed to promote alternative learning outcomes for families with a child recently diagnosed with diabetes. In the study that forms the basis of the model, families felt satisfied with the care and information about diabetes and its treatment they received while they were in hospital, but problems arose when they were discharged. Once home, they felt that what they had learnt was inadequate in the home environment (Wennick 2007). In response, a new care model was designed and tested that is better suited to the various families' daily lives, specifically to improve the families' ability to care for children in a way that maintained good blood sugar control over time. This new evidence-based care model was termed hospital-based home care.[3]

Closely focused on each family's needs, hospital-based home care is a tailored adaptation to lifestyles and habits, designed to help families rapidly and successfully integrate diabetes care into their everyday lives. The defining property of the care model is that it should be possible for families to sustain routines learnt in the initial phase of the disease over the long term. This is achieved by healthcare staff helping parents and children learn on their own terms, rather than by overwhelming them with facts according to a predetermined script. Healthcare professionals have a long tradition of being the experts on how to manage diabetes, but have often operated on the assumption that families will simply follow instructions and adapt their lives to suit the information and advice given. However, patients and families do not always choose to do so; instead, they do what fits their own lifestyle. Hospital-based home care is about trying to improve on this approach so that medical personnel listen to the needs of individual families, and concentrate on supplying the necessary information. Doing so together families and professionals can find a way to manage insulin therapy that both maintains a steady blood sugar level and is within the bounds of reason for the family and child to adapt to (see Hansson in this volume). Hospital-based home care is therefore predicated on families themselves asking for the information they need to manage a range of everyday situations, and learning from others' experiences, putting that information into practice (Tiberg 2012).

What does this new approach demand? It can involve learning how to calculate the right amount of insulin relative to what the children have eaten and how much exercise they have taken that day, how different foods affect the child's blood sugar levels, and how to reverse an episode of low blood sugar. The ambition is that families should stay in hospital no longer than necessary to stabilize the child's blood sugar levels. When they feel ready, they should be given every opportunity to return home to learn how to handle their new situation in a home setting. Hospital-based home care is thus intended to organize healthcare in a way that makes diabetes care more accessible.[4]

The model has been evaluated in a randomized controlled trial by a health science research group, comparing hospital-based home care to existing diabetes care (Tiberg 2012). The study established that the use of hospital-based home care was associated with positive outcomes. Parents were reportedly more satisfied with the information they received, and in addition there were health economic benefits. The study also found that fathers showed a greater, lasting involvement in the child's care. As it was a randomized controlled trial, hospital-based home care thus approaches what in healthcare would be considered an evidence-based model. In other words it is the healthcare model which, based on the available research, could be considered the best suitable paediatric diabetes care practice for those with a new diagnosis.[5] The model can also be said to meet modern healthcare standards, as patients are given greater opportunity to influence their own care (participation) while also being given more responsibility for their own health (self-care) (Nordgren 2009; Alftberg & Hansson 2012). The operation of hospital-based home care can thus be understood as a way of organizing healthcare in a manner that reflects a certain understanding of what modern healthcare is, central to which are opportunities for the rationalization and prioritization of the healthcare sector's finite—and thus limited—resources. In consultation with the research group, the hospital where the study had been conducted decided to proceed with the implementation of hospital-based home care.

When the ambition is to offer patients evidence-based care, it is essential that the care model itself—here, hospital-based home care—with its necessary modifications to organizations and care methods, is translated into care practice. This often requires complex changes to be made to healthcare operations on many different levels. Implementation being a slow process, the changes are unlikely to be immediate or even apparent, and that merely adds to the complexity. The personnel in, say, an endocrinology department first need to be made aware of how they currently handle patients and their relatives, before gradually changing how they go about it. Since it is difficult to change everyday healthcare practices, there is a focus in implementation research on what prevents and promotes change (Rycroft-Malone et al. 2013). The ability to see not only the opportunities, but also the stages and challenges of any implementation process, is crucial to realizing change and improving the care on offer (Nilsson et al 2018).

This chapter is not concerned with the various steps involved in implementation, but rather how the ethnographic method can be used to support the changes that implementation entails.[6] We set out a method with which to identify the less successful implementation processes and the differences of opinion that can otherwise mount up, presenting the organization with challenges. The ethnographic method was applied as two ethnologists—Kristofer Hansson and Gabriella Nilsson—observed healthcare staff meetings where the implementation of hospital-based home care was discussed, while a medical team facilitator—Irén Tiberg—was present to support the process of change. Hansson and Nilsson subsequently observed clinical encounters between medical staff, patients and their relatives.

Diffraction and ethnographic methods

We argue that linking traditional ethnography to the theoretical concept of diffraction (see also Haraway 1988, 1992, 1997; Barad 2007; Johnson 2020) offers a fruitful method with which to examine the implementation processes of evidence-based healthcare practices. The term diffraction is taken from physics, and describes how light, encountering an obstacle, spreads out rather than propagating in a straight line. Similarly, an implementation process can be understood as diffractive, with a variety of understandings made visible during the process. Instead of focusing only on the anticipated and desired processes of change and on the difference that is thereby generated, with the diffractive method the ethnographer can identify the various forms of differentness present (Jackson & Mazzei 2012; Wiszmeg 2017). This differentness is actively evoked when ethnographer and facilitator together problematize the implementation process. The method highlights that knowledge is not a one-sided entity, but rather, as the ethnologist Andréa Wiszmeg notes, something 'highly situational and fluid, with varying durability' (2017, 74).

How, then, to translate the theory into actual practice? There is a risk in assuming the facilitator's task is limited to communicating the care model to the healthcare personnel who are then to change their care practices. Applying the diffraction method, however, makes it possible for the ethnographer to be involved in the various relationships that constitute the implementation process. Through these relationships, we argue, new knowledge can be generated with which to understand the ongoing processes (see also Winther 2017).

Metaphorically, the method can be likened to the ethnographer holding up a lantern in a dark room (Barad 2007, Wiszmeg 2017).[7] In this metaphor, there are two ways for the ethnographer to hold the lantern: holding it still, the light can be used to study the room while moving around; swinging it about, the lantern itself and the play of the light come into focus. The first way to hold the lantern can be compared to traditional ethnography, where the ethnographer studies the cultural expressions that appear in a specific context; the second way makes the lantern—the implementation—the object of the study, not just the means of the study. Swinging the lantern makes it possible to see not only the implementation process, but the various actors' understandings and knowledges of the process.

The lantern's sweep is what results in the dissemination of different knowledge, as Wiszmeg writes:

> This takes into consideration how the participants hold, in a metaphorical way, the ethnographer firmly or loosely, but also what kind of knowledge they gain by doing so and what they can set in motion. If we presuppose a boundary between the ethnographer and the 'other', we should remember that the ethnographer is not only holding, but is also being held. Much like the ethnographer, the 'other' will use the research situation to explore the world surrounding them, together as well as separately. The researcher, too, will be the researched. (Wiszmeg 2017, 76)

From this perspective, not only is there a reflexive approach to the implementation under study, but—or perhaps instead—the ethnographer, together with the facilitator, forms—and evokes—a situated knowledge (Haraway 1988). This is not knowledge in terms of the ethnographer being a neutral observer of an ongoing process, but knowledge arising from situational relationships of which ethnographer and facilitator alike are part. Ethnographically speaking, the diffractive method creates knowledge, which, as Wiszmeg (2017) points out, is the result of both reflection and a disruptive process (see also Mellander & Wiszmeg 2016, 103). Wiszmeg therefore argues that 'It is part of the ethnographers' quest to trace the differences that matter in the subsequent interference patterns' (Wiszmeg 2017, 78).

How can this be done methodologically? In our case the method consisted of many different steps. The ethnographers were present in the initial phase of the process to observe the staff meetings at which the facilitator first presented and discussed the planned implementation. After every meeting, the ethnographers wrote down their observations, and the facilitator read and commented on the texts. Through this reading, a positional shift was made possible where the ethnographers no longer studied a defined object, but together with the facilitator explored the ongoing process of implementation. It is primarily this material that is presented in this chapter. Subsequently, based on joint experiences from the ethnographic material, two interviews were conducted with the facilitator in order to further explore the possibilities and limitations of the implementation—of swinging the lamp rather than holding it still. The entirety of the collected material shows how ethnographers and facilitator together sought new experiences, so increasing the understanding of this particular ongoing implementation process. For the purpose of this chapter, two themes have been selected where these processes were especially evident.

The daily business of implementation

Applying the diffractive ethnographic method, two empirical examples have been selected where the ethnographers and the facilitator together created a new understanding of the implementation process. These examples, representing situations of 'messiness' and 'vagueness', highlight how the facilitator was given the opportunity to actively relate to the processes that had been initiated.

Messiness

The first meetings the facilitator held with the paediatric diabetes care teams that were to implement hospital-based home care, can be viewed as a learning process. This learning process not only included the presentation of a new way of thinking about care and clinical encounters, but was also a negotiation (Fixsen et al. 2005). In order for a sustainable change to come about, it is crucial that from the first there should be an understanding of how and why the change should be implemented, as well as a desire for change (Weiner 2009). For this reason, it is crucial that time is allocated for in-depth discussions between all the personnel involved and the facilitator, and that the latter is being alert to the assumptions and modi operandi that the new evidence-based model might call into question. This matters particularly if the model is likely to challenge working methods that are the basis of the staff's professional identity (Nilsson et al. 2018). Previous research within the project indicates that this is often a very demanding process for the facilitator (Tiberg et al. 2017).

In implementing hospital-based home care, the facilitator began by holding regular information meetings with personnel from two hospital departments (here called Team I and Team II). The teams consisted of different professional categories: paediatricians, paediatric nurses, dieticians and social workers. The aim was both to inform them what the new model would entail in terms of actual care methods and to negotiate a constructive approach to the implementation of the change. At the information meetings, it became clear that staff shortages were felt to be an obstacle to implementation, but equally that staff initially found some of the fundamentals of the model problematic—earlier discharge from hospital, for example. Here it was important that the facilitator gradually changed her way of communicating with the staff in order to mitigate what they saw as ambiguities and contradictions, and to prepare them mentally and emotionally for the changes to come. The latter has been singled out in implementation research as 'readiness for change' (Weiner 2009).

In order for the facilitator to fully relate to what happened at the staff meetings, not only were the ethnographers present as observers, but their resultant ethnographic texts were made available to the facilitator, which she read and annotated. This enabled her to relate to the ethnographic descriptions in the course of the project. The example here is of an observation, commented on by the facilitator, which concerned the departments' prospects for change. At this point, the discussion had turned to staff shortages in the health service in general, and in the departments in particular, as the reason why it was difficult to implement all the changes they wanted to see. Here this change was about one form of patient monitoring they wanted to try in both Team I and Team II:

> The discussion changes direction, and now there is a conversation about staff shortages in the hospital and that staff are finding it

difficult to arrange cover because they are so short-staffed. At the same time, the hospital has imposed a recruitment freeze on all departments and clinics. I was a little unsure about the transition between the various discussions at the meeting, but think it is the senior consultant who changes the topic the group is talking about. Suddenly they are discussing who should do what about the most recent patient monitoring when staff shortages are so severe. It is the senior consultant who drives the discussion, and everyone seemed to agree. One of the nurses tried to solve the immediate practical problem by saying that as she was not working 100 per cent she could increase her hours if it would help. They conclude that there is no solution to be had, but the discussion has at least raised the problem. It is very clear, from my perspective, that Team I is in a difficult situation.

The facilitator's comment upon reading: Spot on—it's like a fog smothering the team's whole being, at the same time as what is said in this discussion is hollow words. The same views have existed the same way for the 13 years I have been in the team, and although the situation has gradually deteriorated and never been as bad as it is now, words have become pretty much mean-ingless. There is a resignedness about it all—we cannot influence the situation but still have to try and find solutions and continue the business of improving.

By being present from the start, the ethnographers had the chance to capture how the discussion about the implementation of hos-pital-based home care was introduced, and what opportunities and limitations the personnel identified. These opportunities and limitations did not necessarily have anything to do with the imple-mentation itself, as seen here, but as readers of this ethnography we could see from the senior consultant's way of describing the shortages of personnel, that theirs was a demanding situation that was unlikely to be made any easier by the team simultaneously having to change the way they worked. That said, in this instance the facilitator was well aware of the situation, and could confirm the ethnographers' observations, putting into words a sequence of events that long predated this specific situation. How did this way of identifying and talking about limitations and opportunities impact on the implementation itself?

First and foremost, this type of diffractive ethnographic observation can problematize the idea that implementation is the 'mainstream of innovation within an organization' (Greenhalgh et al. 2004, 582). 'Mainstream' becomes a metaphor for implementation as a process of change that can be redirected relatively easily, depending on the innovation to be introduced; a metaphor that likens such a process to a stream, and one where it is easy to redirect its flow. However, as much of the literature stresses, healthcare is noted for its 'messiness' (Woolf 2008; Hertzum et al. 2017). This messiness, we argue, must be addressed in any implementation process. Though messiness too, obviously, is a metaphor, it is a metaphor that shows the opposite: what is running counter to what is expected or not working at all; what is refusing all attempts to redirect it or is redirected far too quickly.

The facilitator, together with the observing ethnographers, could make the processes of implementation visible in a way that either strengthened the centripetal 'mainstream' forces or actively try to relate to what is collectively defined as its 'messiness'. By choosing the latter situated knowledges of various kinds were constructed, that would help with other approaches when the facilitator next met the group. The ethnographic text is not only a way to make the things the facilitator cannot see or relate to visible, but it also confirms the facilitator's existing perspectives, which might need some thought.

In looking for alterative perspectives on the implementation—creating fresh contextual understandings together—one of the ethnographers chose to conduct interviews with the facilitator, in part to go over the facilitator's comments on the ethnography. By doing so, they arrived at further situated interpretations to apply to the ongoing implementation process. The ethnographer reading the facilitator's annotations, quoted above, aloud, preceded this section of the interview:

Facilitator: There is a helplessness.

Ethnographer: There is a helplessness to this. We cannot influence the situation, but we still have to try to find solutions. Continue with the changes. But then it's…

Facilitator: It's really difficult. It really is.

Ethnographer: But it's down to the entire hospital management. That's all you see in the media … healthcare scandal.

Facilitator: And we're powerless in the face of it. A bit dejected. I think so. We are a bit dejected by it actually.

Ethnographer: But for Team II it's … even though it's the same hospital [after a reorganization], they're a bit better off … or is it the same for them?

Facilitator: Well it's because last autumn… Team I is a slightly larger team than Team II, and we've had two full-time diabetes nurses in each. I used to be one of the ones in Department I. In Department II there was the diabetes nurse who was one of the first diabetes nurses in Sweden. A tower of strength, such a support … She's been an incredibly important member of their team in Department II. She retired in the autumn and then the resources for the diabetes nurses halved. […] Which means this spring the resources for the diabetic nurses have been thin on the ground. When it comes to doctors too things are really tight. So all told, this spring the staffing situation has been truly awful. […] It's a major obstacle, and at the same time so you're powerless. Oh yes, we're working on it, and the idea is that soon things will be back to us having two full-time positions. There's something going on behind the scenes that we don't really know about. I feel a bit as if you have to try to look past it and do what we can in the meanwhile.

Together, the ethnographer and facilitator help find a form of interchange which gives them an idea of the current situation in Team I and II. By holding the lantern together, they create an understanding of what is going on in the background, behind the actual implementation process. This means not only that the ethnographer has a better idea of what is going on in the implementation process, but that the facilitator has the chance to get new insights about the process of change that is underway—putting feelings into words and finding different explanations for them. It does not have to be limited to things that are already known if not understood, however, as the method can also be used to make previously invisible processes visible.

Vagueness

The facilitator was not always aware of exactly what she had communicated at staff meetings, but rather, as the second example shows, it became clear when she read the ethnography afterwards. This not only made any issues visible, but also put them into words. The following ethnography illustrates the course of events:

> The facilitator mentions that the project can be seen as individualized care and in the same breath says that this is 'a bit vague', I have no idea what she means by vague. Is she referring to some general context at this particular workplace which means individualized care has been seen as being vague? Or is it that she wants somehow to reduce the value of her own study, that it'd make it too important in relation to all the problems they're facing now, such as the staff shortage? It's crucial to avoid pop psychology, but the connection between vagueness and individualized care says something about how a project is presented.
>
> Facilitator's written comment upon reading: Given your reaction I am embarrassed by my choice of words, and at the same time very grateful to be able to read it. The reason I use the word is that I think (and have heard lots of times too) that individualized is felt to be very abstract and nobody really knows what it means. One standard comment is that's what we do already. I use the word because I think I take some key people with me as they are (diabetic nurses and to some extent even doctors) by using their terminology. The majority of these people have heard me present the study findings several times, and the term 'individu-

alized care' is a central concept. Every time I talk about this with people in the teams, I try to find other ways of expressing myself so that they can see or understand the meaning of the concept.

The facilitator went on to list the advantages of the new care method to be implemented—better blood sugar levels, beneficial for the children discharged to go home, happier children and families, and it all costs less—and here the emphasis was no longer on the 'messiness' of healthcare, but rather on the way the facilitator presented the key features of the new hospital-based home care model. As an ethnographer, it is possible to observe not only what is said, but also the context in which it was said and how people react to it, both physically and verbally. By drawing up a detailed account of the process, it becomes possible for the facilitator to revisit and reflect on the situation later.

Implementation that focuses too much on the mainstream metaphor risks accounting for the process in an overly simplistic fashion where, for example, the facilitator can relatively easily communicate an evidence-based care model to the personnel who are to put it into action. In research, knowledge is often talked about in terms of knowledge translation, as just such one-way communication (Engelbretsen et al. 2017). Yet as the example above makes plain, there is not necessarily so simple a transfer when hospital-based home care is 'translated' from one individual to the next in real life; rather, it is a complex process, coloured by both the facilitator's own approach to the implementation of hospital-based home care, and the sense healthcare professionals make of what is said at staff meetings of the kind described here.

In the interview, this formulation is a topic of some discussion between the ethnographer and the facilitator. Further layers of interpretation were added to how the facilitator could relate to the ongoing implementation process. As the facilitator said,

> My aim is they should see or understand the meaning of the term [individualized care]. Because when you read it like this, that word

sounds utterly stupid. As you wrote … introducing individual-ized care … well, it's just vague. So that I realize it doesn't seem very professional. My focus is always to try to meet the people in that room where they are. I don't think it's such an odd choice of word for them, actually. […] So, you've got something that's very abstract and you don't understand, and you… I sometimes feel that there is a genuine interest, actually, if you only knew how. But you don't know how. So I reckon this is definitely harder. We've come back to it several times. How can I somehow contribute to this change of attitude?

The facilitator ultimately asks the most important question—how can she drive the changes needed for the implementation process. With ethnography, it is possible to make this process visible *and* to reflect on it afterwards. It is this reflective work that offers oppor-tunities to create situated knowledge together of a kind that can alter the ongoing process. The ethnographers draw one form of understanding from the actual observation, and another form—or multiple forms—when the facilitator comments on events by annotating the ethnographic texts. When they then talk through the observations and the facilitator's written comments, a further form of situated knowledge is achieved. Here knowledge is not just something that is in circulation at staff meetings, but which all parties involved must work with far more actively throughout the implementation process, creating situated knowledge together on a variety of occasions, in the realization that such varieties of knowledge are a way forward. How the facilitator was affected on each occasion, and how the varieties of situated knowledge fed back into the implementation process, are things that are harder to quantify retrospectively. The point of this chapter is to explore how an approach in which a facilitator and ethnographers work closely together might further the implementation of a new care method, but at the same time their collaboration amounts to an important ethnographic fact, which can be adduced in the cultural analysis of the implementation process.

Conclusions

With changes to a variety of healthcare practices, the implementation of evidence-based models has become increasingly common. Implementation can be understood as the process by which a care model—in this instance, hospital-based home care—translates into a new care method, but it is also a theoretical perspective which concentrates on how change transpires. The purpose of this chapter has been to show that such changes are often opaquely complex, which gives weight to the argument that continued in-depth research on implementation processes is needed. What should be singled out is the importance of research that focuses on the significance of context—or organizational culture, if one prefers—in whether or not an implementation process will lead to sustainable change.

The chapter explores the possibilities open to ethnographers and facilitators to band together to create situated knowledge that can benefit the implementation process. The term diffraction is suggested as a possible method with which to generate a variety of situated knowledges during a process (Haraway 1997; Barad 2007; Wiszmeg 2017). Just two examples have been discussed here, but the working method is unlimited in scope, and a wide variety of themes could result from joint efforts of this kind.

One finding is the way in which the various processes are best understood. Three different perspectives on knowledge are apparent, each of which brings home the full complexity of implementation, and shows how the proposed method can be understood in relation to processes of knowledge and change in general—from evidence-based knowledge, via care models and care practices, to situated knowledge:

(*i*) In a contemporary perspective on healthcare, scientific, so-called evidence-based knowledge is evidently a primary category—knowledge with capital K. When it comes to healthcare research, this knowledge can best be described in terms of a model for practice, here a care model. In this chapter, hospital-based home care is the care model implemented.

(*ii*) For evidence-based knowledge to be operationalized, the resultant care model must be reframed as a care method, adapted to the specific care context in which the model will be applied. This translation process can vary in problematics or scope, depending on the readiness and willingness to change. Regardless, there is inevitably a point at which the different care methods meet—the method supported by the model and the method (the professional knowledge) already in operation in the healthcare context—which here was hospital-based home care and the traditional hospital care. The reason for the implementation is to replace the previous care method with the new evidence-based method. In order for this to be successful, we would argue that it is necessary to think not in terms of replacing traditional care outright, but rather to try to achieve a coalition of the two methods in what we have termed situated knowledge.

(*iii*) By using the method we propose here, where the ethnographers and facilitator work diffractively, knowledge is generated which draws on both the evidence-based model and the professional knowledge already found in the context of the new model's implementation. It is co-created knowledge that combines all the evidence, with its potential outcomes, in the specific context where it is implemented.

Diffractive ethnography is largely reliant on ethnographers daring to abandon their personal reflexive interpretations—which easily create a distance to the study object (Barad 2007; Wiszmeg 2017)—to meet the person being studied partway in a joint interpretation. Together they hold the lantern so that the facilitator, the other, becomes an important factor in the way situated knowledge is generated, influencing the processes of change that are already underway by the simple act of seeing them.

Notes

1 We wish to thank Andréa Wiszmeg for her comments on earlier drafts of this chapter.

2 Implementation research identifies four main factors as having an impact on implementation: (*i*) innovation; (*ii*) how innovation is communicated; (*iii*) time; and (*iv*) the sociocultural system in which innovation is implemented (Rogers 2003).

3 Our account of the implementation process enlarges on our previous publication 'Att implementera tillgänglighet i vården' ('Implementing accessibility in healthcare') in Hansson & Nilsson 2017.

4 The Swedish Health and Medical Services Act of 2017 (Hälso- och sjukvårdslagen 2017:30) said of accessibility that 'Healthcare must be provided so that the requirements for good care are met. This means that care in particular should be readily accessible.'

5 At the same time, it is important to acknowledge that a single study does not constitute a sufficient basis, but together with other research with similar findings the evidence becomes stronger. Central to this are proven experience and a consensus among the professionals who provide the care that children will do best in a home environment as far as possible. The crucial question is thus whether it is safe for a child newly diagnosed with type 1 diabetes to be at home rather than in hospital. This was a source of anxiety for some of the nursing staff who were to work with hospital-based home care, and led some to resist its implementation (discussed in greater detail in Nilsson et al. 2018).

6 The implementation process can in theory be broken down into different steps, from preparatory work to full implementation as a sustainable practice. In brief, they can be said to be (*i*) installation, (*ii*) initial implementation, and (*iii*) full implementation. This chapter is based on the division of the implementation process presented in the survey 'Implementation Research: A Synthesis of the Literature' (Fixsen et al. 2005; see also Rogers 2003).

7 We draw on Andréa Wiszmeg's reading (2017) of Karen Michelle Barad's philosophy where Barad's stick becomes a lantern, linking it to an older ethnological trope of the searchlight (see Daun 2010). As Barad says of her metaphor, 'One need only remember here the sensation, often cited by psychologists, which every one has experienced when attempting to orient himself in a dark room with a stick. When the stick is held loosely, it appears to the sense of touch to be an object. When, however, it is held firmly, we lose the sensation that it is a foreign body, and the impression of touch becomes immediately localized at the point where the stick is touching the body under investigation' (2007, 154).

References

Alftberg, Åsa & Kristofer Hansson (2012), 'Introduction: Self-care translated into practice', *Culture Unbound: Journal of Current Cultural Research*, 4, 415–24.

Ashmore, Malcolm (1989), *The reflexive thesis: Writing sociology of scientific knowledge* (Chicago: Univ. of Chicago Press).

Barad, Karen Michelle (2007), *Meeting the universe halfway: Quantum physics and the entanglement of matter and meaning* (Durham: Duke University Press).

Barrett, Susan M. (2004), 'Implementation studies: Time for a revival? Personal reflections on 20 years of implementation studies', *Public Administration*, 82(2), 249–62.

Bohlin, Ingemar & Morten Sager (2011) (eds.), *Evidensens många ansikten: Evidensbaserad praktik i praktiken* (Lund: Arkiv Förlag).

Bragesjö, Fredrik (2004), *Praktiserad reflexivitet: En vetenskapsteoretisk studie av forskningspolitisk forskning och vetenskapssociologi* (diss., Gothenburg: Göteborgs universitet).

Daun, Åke (2010), *Med rörligt sökarljus: Den nya etnologins framväxt under 1960- och 1970-talen* (Stockholm: Dejavu).

Engelbretsen, Eivind, Tony Joakim Sandset & John Ødemark (2017), 'Expanding the knowledge translation metaphor', *Health Research Policy & Systems*, 15(19).

Fixsen, D. L., S. F. Naoom, K. A. Blase, R. M. Friedman & F. Wallace (2005), *Implementation research: A synthesis of the literature* (National Implementation Research Network (FMHI) Publication, 231; Tampa, FL: Louis de la Parte Florida Mental Health Institute, University of South Florida).

Greenhalgh, T., G. Robert, F. Macfarlane, P. Bate & O. Kyriakidou (2004), 'Diffusion of innovations in service organizations: Systematic review and recommendations', *Milbank Quarterly*, 82(4), 581–629.

Hansson, Kristofer & Gabriella Nilsson (2017), 'Att implementera tillgänglighet i vården', in Lars Nordgren (ed.), *Health management: Att göra hälso- och sjukvård mer tillgänglig* (Stockholm: Sanoma Utbildning).

Haraway, Donna Jeanne (1988), 'Situated knowledges: The science question in feminism and the privilege of partial perspective', *Feminist Studies*, 14(3), 575–99.

—— (1992), *The promises of monsters: A regenerative politics for inappropriate/d others* (New York: Routledge).

—— (1997), *Modest_Witness@Second_Millennium. FemaleMan™_Meets_OncoMouse©: Feminism and technoscience* (New York: Routledge).

Hertzum, Morten, Maria le Manikas & Arnvør á Torkilsheyggi (2017), 'Grappling with the future: The messiness of pilot implementation in information systems design', *Health Informatics Journal*, 25(2), 372–88.

Jackson, Alecia Youngblood & Lisa A. Mazzei (2012), *Thinking with theory in qualitative research: Viewing data across multiple perspectives* (New York: Routledge).

Johnson, Ericka (2020), *Refracting through technologies: Bodies, medical technologies and norms* (London: Routledge).

Law, John (1996), 'Pensamiento Traduction/Trahison: Notes on ANT', *Convergencia*, 13(42).

Mellander, Elias & Andréa Wiszmeg (2016), 'Interfering with others: Re-configuring ethnography as a diffractive practice', *Kulturstudier*, 93–115.

Mol, Annemarie (1999), 'Ontological politics: A word and some questions', in John Law & John Hassard (eds.), *Actor network theory and after* (Oxford: Blackwell).

—— (2002), *The body multiple: Ontology in medical practice* (Durham: Duke University Press).

Nilsson, Gabriella, Kristofer Hansson, Irén Tiberg & Inger Hallström (2018), 'How dislocation and professional anxiety influence readiness for change during the implementation of hospital-based home care for children newly diagnosed with diabetes—An ethnographic analysis of the logic of workplace change', *BMC Health Services research*, 18, 1–10.

Nordgren, Lars (2009), 'Value creation in health care services—Developing service productivity: Experiences from Sweden', *International Journal of Public Sector Management*, 22(2), 114–27.

Richards, David A. & Ingalill Rahm Hallberg (2015) (eds.), *Complex interventions in health: An overview of research methods* (Abingdon: Routledge).

Rogers, Everett M. (2003), *Diffusion of innovations* (New York: Free Press).

Rycroft-Malone, J., K. Seers, J. Chandler, C. A. Hawkes, N. Crichton, C. Allen, I. Bullock & L. Strunin (2013), 'The role of evidence, context, and facilitation in an implementation trial: Implications for the development of the PARIHS framework', *Implementation Science*, 8, 1–13.

Saetren, Harald (2005), 'Facts and myths about research on public policy implementation: Out-of-fashion, allegedly dead, but still very much alive and relevant', *Policy Studies Journal*, 33(4), 559–82.

Svensk sjuksköterskeförening (2016), 'Evidensbaserad vård och omvårdnad' (Stockholm: Svensk sjuksköterskeförening. https://www.swenurse.se/globalassets/01-svensk-sjuk-skoterskeforening/publikationer-svensk-sjukskoterskeforening/ssf-om-publikationer/svensk.sjukskoterskeforening.ssf.om.evidensbasera.vard_2016_2016_webb.pdf

Tiberg, Irén (2012), *The initial care when a child is diagnosed with type 1 diabetes* (diss., Lund: Faculty of Medicine, Lund University).

—— Kristofer Hansson, Robert Holmberg & Inger Hallström (2017), 'An ethnographic observation study of the facilitator role in an implementation process', *BMC Research Notes*, 10.

Weiner, B. J. (2009), 'A theory of organizational readiness for change', *Implementation Science*, 4(67).

Wennick, Anne (2007), *Living with childhood diabetes: Family experiences and long-term effects* (diss., Lund: Faculty of Medicine, Lund University).

WHO (2006), 'Bridging the "know–do" gap. Meeting on knowledge translation in global health' (WHO/EIP/KMS/2006.2; Geneva: WHO). https://www.measureevaluation.org/resources/training/capacity-building-resources/high-impact-research-training-curricula/bridging-the-know-do-gap.pdf

Winther, Jonas (2017), *Making it work: Trial work between scientific elegance and everyday life workability* (Copenhagen: Det Humanistiske Fakultet, Københavns Universitet).

—— (2017), 'Diffractions of the foetal cell suspension: Scientific knowledge and value in laboratory work', in Kristofer Hansson & Markus Idvall (eds.), *Interpreting the brain in society: Cultural reflections on neuroscientific practices* (Lund: Arkiv).

Woolf, Steven H. (2008), 'The meaning of translational research and why it matters', *JAMA*, 299(2), 211–13.

Woolgar, Steve (1988) (ed.), *Knowledge and reflexivity: New frontiers in the sociology of knowledge* (London: Sage).

PART IV

KNOWLEDGE IN EVERYDAY EXPERIENCE

CHAPTER 7

A number in circulation

HbA1c as standardized knowledge in diabetes care

Kristofer Hansson

A glycosylated haemoglobin test, HbA1c, is a blood test that measures how much sugar is bound to the red blood cells, or haemoglobin (Hb). Since red blood cells break down after about 120 days and new ones are formed, HbA1c can be used to check the average blood sugar over the last two to three months, and thus how a patient is managing their diabetes. If the patient's blood sugar levels have been good, less sugar will be attached to the haemoglobin. On 1 September 2010, HbA1c tests in Sweden were changed from being given as a percentage to being given in mmol/mol. As a result, patients' HbA1c results became comparable, not only individually, but also across cohorts of patients, and as an average value for regions and the entire country. It even became internationally comparable between countries. In other words, HbA1c tests circulated on an entirely new scale and took on various meanings in relation to the diagnosis of diabetes. In this chapter, HbA1c is investigated as a form of standardized knowledge in diabetes care and the significance this form of knowledge has for a variety of practices is explored. HbA1c is discussed here as a value expressed in figures, but where the figures are interpreted, translated, and understood—enacted—in different ways, depending on the practice presenting or using the figures. Ethnographic methods allow us to follow the figures and how they are discussed, whether at staff meetings or in individual clinical encounters with parents whose children have recently been diagnosed with diabetes. These are figures which can serve as a key metric in the narrative that professionals create in the clinical encounter, a narrative that emphasizes the importance of managing one's diabetes (Arduser 2017). It can also be a narrative that visualizes developments at an endocrinology department in a national comparison with other departments' averages for HbA1c. However, the representation of figures produced by HbA1c testing is not limited to narratives or visualizations, but is used for a wide range of quantifications, measurements, and standardizations according to the subject— doctor, nurse, patient, parent, and so on (see Larsen & Røyrvik 2017). In other words, it forms the normative guidelines to which various subjects relate differently—it is a conditional circulation.

This chapter explores how figures are used in medicine to create normative guidelines, and how figures are variously interpreted and used depending on the contextual practice. I begin by presenting HbA1c and the study's methods and implementation, and then trace the figures from the clinical encounters to staff meetings, all in a Swedish welfare context.[1] Clinical encounters establish the significance of the figures for the interaction of medical staff and children with diabetes and their families. This practice is then compared to how the professionals discuss and use HbA1c at staff meetings, and how this relates to a national context, which sees medical professionals use the figures to compare themselves with other endocrinology departments. The chapter concludes by addressing not only how HbA1c creates figures which are in constant circulation, but also by examining the subjectification processes in which the individual becomes 'diabetic' by the use of these figures and others (see Agamben 2014). In the next section I begin the chapter by addressing the question of the realities where these specific figures—these dispositifs—apply.

The all-important figure of 52

A dispositif is a theoretical concept that renders visible the relations that arise when a harmless object such as HbA1c is put into practice, creating a network of power relations between, say, a medical institution and the individual (see Agamben 2014). It is in the meeting of individual and dispositif—here, HbA1c—that the subject proclaims itself, be they doctor, nurse, patient, or relative. This assertion was something I saw in one of the many staff meetings I attended which brought together all the department's specialists to discuss, on this occasion, a leaflet about HbA1c for families whose children have diabetes. There were nearly twenty people seated at a long table, mainly doctors and nurses, but also dieticians, counsellors, psychologists, and medical secretaries, who together made up the hospital's diabetes team. Most of them fetched mugs of coffee or tea, and, having agreed on the agenda, began by discussing the leaflet.

One of the key points in the leaflet was that 'Your diabetes treatment goal' was an HbA1c of 52 mmol/mol.[2] This was a test done when the patient attended the hospital clinic; it was not something the child or their family could measure on their own.[3] To achieve this goal, the diabetic child had to keep their blood sugar at a low level. The leaflet therefore spelt out these levels, with, for example, 'Blood sugar before a meal: 4–6 mmol/l' and 'Target value at bedtime 5–7 mmol/l'.[4] If the family arranged everyday life practices so the child's blood sugar remained within these averages, then the chances of achieving the HbA1c target of 52 mmol/mol increased. In order to achieve this the leaflet had a section with 'Help reaching your goals', which began with 'Test your blood sugar before every meal!' followed by 'Hypoglycaemia', 'Correction dose', 'Counting carbs', and 'Exercise'. These points summed up the hope that the family would take responsibility not only for the child's treatment, but also for reaching their health goals with a form of self-care (Alftberg & Hansson 2012; Arduser 2017; Liu and Lundin in this volume).

What was this self-care that the parents or patient were expected to manage? *Hypoglycaemia* is when blood sugar falls below 3.5–4 mmol/l, which the individual should treat with glucose to raise their blood sugar. If their blood sugar is above 8 mmol/l then they need to take a *correction dose* of insulin, and their blood sugar should be checked again after two hours. Family and teenage patients should learn to *count carbs*, adjusting the insulin dose according to how many carbohydrates there are in the meal the patient will eat and what physical activity is planned afterwards. By looking at both, the family can 'estimate how much insulin is needed for a certain quantity of carbohydrates'. It is thus not a question of there being a fixed dose of insulin to take, but rather a form of self-care in which the family calculates the correct dose of insulin. When it comes to *exercise*, the leaflet pointed out that 'Physical activity will help you reach your goal. Regular exercise will help keep your blood sugar stable and you will feel better in both the short and the long term!' This information imposes a dispositif on the family that not only creates a relation to the 'standardized knowledge' of healthcare (Agamben 2014), but also makes visible the knowledge subject who has experience enough to practise self-care (Foucault 1978; Alftberg & Hansson 2012).

At the staff meeting, the first person to talk about the leaflet was one of the doctors, Emma, who wanted to stress it was very useful, because it gave the family information about HbA1c and because 'patients are happier for taking something with them' when leaving the clinic (meaning that most families of children with newly diagnosed diabetes liked having both verbal and written information). One of the other doctors, Anders, objected, noting that 'At the same time they get the diabetes book, and that says that you should not obsess about HbA1c'. Emma believed that the perspective in the diabetes book was incorrect, and she had a different experience from her clinical encounters, namely that the need for information about HbA1c varied from family to family: 'Good to have it on paper, but it's individual.' By way of example, she talked about a family where the parents had separated and 'don't know which way they're facing': for them, the target values in the leaflet were a help. The goals were something the parents could agree on, and set the tone in both households for how the two should manage their child's diabetes. Kerstin, one of the older doctors, pointed out that HbA1c risked 'being judge and jury' for families who, not as successful at managing their child's disease, had readings well above the target value of 52 mmol/mol. Many around the table wanted to comment on this—plainly, Kerstin's statement was the sort that elicited differing opinions. Some said there was a risk of creating 'neurotic parents and patients' because of all the endless calculations they would have to do to reach an HbA1c of 52 or below. Emma defended her position, once again referring to the families who were happy with the information by saying that 'many people think it's comforting'. Kerstin qualified her earlier statement by saying it was important that they 'never hand out the document without saying how it should be used', and finished by saying 'one must discuss it'.

This ethnographic description of how the leaflet was discussed by medical professionals shows that HbA1c is not value-neutral. Instead, it comes down to a figure linked to medical treatment guidelines, which are understood and interpreted according to the practices of the healthcare professionals at the staff meeting. The medical staff fell into at least two camps. One welcomed parents and children being given information about how they should manage their treatment in their everyday lives to reach an HbA1c of 52 mmol/mol. They pointed out that parents and older children could aim for this with regular blood sugar monitoring, counting carbohydrates before taking insulin, and encouraging exercise. Under those circumstances the HbA1c test taken when the family attended the hospital clinic would not be an abstract value, but rather could be an acknowledgment that the family had success-fully treated the child's diabetes on a daily basis. Given this, we can better understand Emma's statement that 'it's comforting' for parents to know about the target value and that it is worth trying to reach it. The professionals who objected to the leaflet felt that the focus on figures, insulin doses, carbohydrates, and exercise meant that the illness featured too prominently in family life. This is not immediately evident from this ethnographic description, but it was an enduring topic of discussion at staff meetings where the healthcare professionals looked at diabetes care. There were parents and patients, they said, who overdid the counting and became 'neurotic', forgetting to carry on living their lives as before the diagnosis.[5] The attitude was that today's advanced diabetes treatment should not only reduce the long-term sequelae, but can also enable families to continue living much as before. Some felt that an HbA1c of 52 mmol/mol could be felt by families and children to be casting blame, instead of encouraging them to work with medical staff to become better at managing the disease.

A central feature of the discussion was how the medical professionals used the figure of 52 in certain ways to argue for their views of diabetes care. The figure thus took on different meanings. Was it a figure parents and patients should strive to attain, or was it a figure that should be hidden away and not talked about in clinical encounters? Was it only of relevance to medical staff, or should families and children be told it was a target value? There is no easy answer to these questions; as we will see, the different uses are reliant on the data to accord to the practice. At the staff meeting, the figure was an opportunity for individuals to position themselves on how they as professionals related to the treatment of diabetes. The figure was not simply a figure, but also a naming practice that made the world intelligible to the professionals (Eliassen 2008). The professionals could talk about the parents and patients as those who reached the target and those who failed and thus needed more help from the healthcare system. There was the latitude to include in this the 'neurotic' families who were too controlling of their children. Whose attempts to manage the disease had an adverse effect on family life, and similarly to reflect on the clinical encounter and that some patients and families felt the figure was 'judge and jury' on whether they had taken responsibility for their child's self-care. The figure allowed them to pigeonhole families and patients they met in clinical encounters into what amounted to a naming practice.

Gunhild Tøndel argues there are two naming processes, where the one seen here is to use figures to name and identify *things* (2017). HbA1c enables medical staff to identify patients, in the same way that patients and their families can relate to it as a value—a form of subjectification process (Agamben 2014). In the second of Tøndel's naming processes it gives each patient an identity, and can thus follow their development using the figure. Here the name is a tool that enables social and material organization (Tøndel 2017). By taking an HbA1c test every time the patient attends the clinic, it becomes possible to monitor each patient's progress. This is a form of the desubjectification process: it is nearly impossible for the family and the patient to avoid the dispositif, and instead they are subject to HbA1c's specific way of ordering reality (Agamben 2014).

The HbA1c test thus generates categorizations, embodied in figures that differentiate between values—values thought of as good for patient health versus values thought to have a negative impact on patient health. The categorizations are also central to the interaction between the subject and the figures (Hacking 1999). In the ethnography above, this interaction took the form of positioning, as the various professions—the doctors primarily—chose how to relate to the blood test, which resulted not only in their differing approaches to HbA1c, but also in that interaction being placed front and centre in the clinical encounter. The categories impact how the subject perceives and acts in daily life—in the lifeworld (Husserl 2002)—but at the same time they serve as exclusionary mechanisms by ensuring that one interaction takes place but not another, so creating standardized knowledge which, depending on the practice, has a claim to power (Foucault 1993).[6] As described in the ethnography above, it was the doctors who positioned themselves most strongly and used their standardized medical knowledge of HbA1c to express their views on the best diabetes care, which came down to a choice between providing families and patients with a great deal of information or limiting it somewhat. We can thus follow HbA1c as a test of a range of practices, charting how standardized knowledge generated by the figures takes on different meanings according to how those figures are used. One central practice in healthcare is the clinical encounter, but before studying how HbA1c is mediated and negotiated—or used, I will turn to the study's methods and materials.

Follow the numbers

Ethnographic descriptions have been used to follow medical *things* in a variety of practices (Prout 1996; Whyte et al. 2002). In the present study HbA1c is just such a thing, which we can follow and describe as it is produced, used, and transformed in different situations. These descriptions use a wide range of ethnographic methods, and generate a multifaceted material with which to capture the full complexity of HbA1c (Marcus 1995). The study is largely based on observations, but such methods as observation-based conversations and document analysis were also used.

Ethnographic observations require the researcher to be present in the setting to be studied, and to record the specific context by describing in words the course of events and settings. An example of this kind of ethnographic description is given above. It is by the researcher's presence it becomes possible to not only describe how figures are presented and discussed, but also how they are used, interpreted, rejected, problematized, promoted, or ignored. Frequently this is hard to capture, because those involved do not necessarily reflect on the process or because it happens unconsciously; being present, observing, gives the ethnographer a greater chance to observe, which is not always possible with interviews or questionnaires (Frykman & Gilje 2003; Ehn & Löfgren 2010). It is central to the method that the researcher is present on different occasions, in order to then compare and problematize the observations. In this study, this comparative perspective is used to analyse how figures circulated and acquired different meanings depending on the practice.

Presence is a particular feature of the ethnographic method, and results in a unique empirical material that would not have been possible if the researcher had not been present, observing. The corollary is that the material is coloured by the researcher's gaze and powers of observation. In this chapter, this is evident in occasional moments of self-reflection when the researcher's position becomes visible (Beckman 2009). This positioning is crucial in order to identify the circumstances of the observation and subsequent analysis. While this empiricism may appear subjective, the unique source material is invaluable for highlighting and problematizing cultural processes which are non-standard in medical and health-care research (Skott 2013).

Five staff meetings, similar to the one described in the passage above, were observed in the space of eight months. Some meetings were quite brief—over in an hour and a half—while others were longer and took a whole morning or afternoon. As the researcher I sat at the table, but to one side, and I avoided joining in the conversation. The professionals' conversations and actions were observed and written down in a notebook, and immediately after each observation the notes were assembled in a digital observation text about ten pages long. I also attached the documents that the group's professionals had produced or discussed on that occasion, whether the medical staff's working papers or information leaflets for patients and parents. Before and after the meetings I chatted with the staff, thus forming relationships that coloured my impression of them as individuals and as a group. Some of them I came to know in their professional roles, and in that way they became key informants, helping me understand the healthcare system better.

Another class of source material is the clinical encounter. For the present study I followed seven families, all with children recently diagnosed with diabetes, who had therefore been admitted to hospital on a fairly urgent basis. Treatment had fallen to the parents almost immediately—with the child participating if in late teenage years—and after a few days they could return home, initially on day release, but soon sleeping at home. After a week or so, the patient was discharged, but with a referral to the hospital clinic for follow-up care and regular check-ups. In most cases, as researcher I entered the picture a few days after their first emergency admission to hospital, and I followed the family for three or four weeks. I was present for a number of their clinical encounters, seated quietly in the background, recording the conversation and associated events. The resultant observation notes formed the basis of the observation texts. These varied in length because the number of observations was different for each family; they range from ten to twenty pages of computer-written text. For each clinical encounter, I always arrived with the medical staff in the hospital department where the family were waiting. In the clinic, I rarely spoke to families in the waiting room, and instead remained with the doctor or the nurse. I deliberately avoided striking up a social relationship with the families or their children, having chosen this approach to my informants because the study is primarily focused on the healthcare professionals' daily lives, not on parents' or children's experiences of diabetes care.

The study was approved in advance by an ethical board, and besides complying with the principles of research ethics the fieldwork was discussed at length with colleagues during the project. This is a sensitive area of study, and the researcher must always consider the special situations that can arise when people meet in healthcare settings such as clinical encounters. It is not enough in an ethnographic study to conduct an ethical review; the researcher must maintain an ethical approach throughout, endeavouring to see the individual—the subject—and understand their situation (Hansson 2013; Fioretos et al. 2013). If nothing else, this approach lends itself to fieldwork, where researchers must be quick to adapt to any situation. This was also the reason I chose to follow the medical staff, leaving it to them to be the first to meet the patient and the family, and why I was always careful to be in the background in clinical encounters. All those involved have been anonymized for this chapter, and any identifiable personal characteristics removed.

Figures in clinical encounters

When Annemarie Mol (2002) followed hospital cases of atherosclerosis to study how bodies with the disease are not just specific actors as described in, for example, patient information, she found instead there were a variety of explanations when the diagnosis and the diseased body met in the clinical encounter, when doctors spoke at conferences, when testing and diagnosing patients, and so on. To capture this complexity, she suggests the concept of *the body multiple*; a very useful approach to understanding how different bodies are created by the healthcare system, depending on the practice. The term does not necessarily equate with a fragmentation of healthcare or a life with a disease, but rather that varying practices arise depending on the situation where diagnosis, body, and disease become visible, as something for all actors to relate to.

Much of the bodies' visibility is achieved with the figures found in the healthcare system's many practices. The figures are co-creators of the bodies that materialize when the patient undergoes the tests to generate data with which to make diagnoses and prognoses (Gadamer 1996). The patient's body could be one with good test values—good figures—and thus the individual or family is praised by the staff for managing their treatment properly. It might be that they show the patient's health is failing, whereupon another type of body results, one which must be corrected. The figures thus have the character of things that can either disregard the body or bring it sharply into focus when the figures bode ill (Heidegger 2013; Agamben 2014).[7] The following ethnographic examples from one clinical encounter demonstrate this interaction, and how a single consultation can feature the body multiple.

The clinical encounter in question was a consultation with a doctor and a nurse at a diabetes clinic by a mother and father and their 4-year-old son. The boy had been diagnosed with diabetes a few weeks before, and the family had recently returned home and were now trying to fit diabetes treatment into their normal lives. The boy had gone back to preschool, but his mother was at home with him the rest of the time. The consultation began with the nurse showing them how to download the blood sugar data from the boy's glucometer, which stores the readings taken by the family. The computer for this was out in the waiting room, and in future the staff expected them to do the download on their own before the doctor saw them, but the parents had yet to learn because it was their first time at the clinic since their son had been admitted to hospital. After the data was transferred, the nurse took the boy and his parents to a test room to do an HbA1c test. The nurse turned to the parents to say, 'He'll have a lower HbA1c than when he came in sick.' By stressing that the diagnosis had a before and an after, the nurse implied there were two bodies even before she did the test: when the parents took the boy to hospital there was the sick body that needed urgent care, and now after a few weeks of treatment here was this body, with its more stable blood sugar levels. This distinction was to recur in the clinical encounter, it being fundamental to this disease, because the patient will always have diabetes and so will always have to manage the treatment.

The parents did not comment on the nurse's remark, and instead the mother asked a question that seemed to be on her mind: at what point should they, the parents, check whether the boy has ketones. The nurse began by explaining what ketones are—the product of the breakdown of fatty acids, a substance the body forms when there is a lack of insulin or if the patient has taken too little insulin. Too many ketones will make a patient ill, and so-called ketone poisoning is life-threatening. To answer the mother's question, she added that they could 'try checking some time with a pee stick'. The mother wondered 'How?' and the nurse explained how to do it by holding the stick under the stream of urine for a second—but 'don't dip it into pee'. She also pointed out how important it was to do the test whenever the boy had an upset stomach or was vomiting to rule out ketone poisoning, because the symptoms are the same. After this exchange there was suddenly another body in the test room, a body which could become acutely ill, requiring the parents to act quickly and drive the child to A & E.

Suddenly, the machine measuring the HbA1c beeped, and the nurse said '55' aloud so the parents could hear. The mother said immediately, 'But that's not 52.' The nurse responded by saying, 'But on the right track.' Previous consultations when they were staying on the ward, together with the paperwork they had been given by the staff, had impressed on the family they needed to get the boy's HbA1c down to 52 mmol/mol, so it was not surprising that the mother reacted as she did: 55 was a value she felt was a failure. Yet as the nurse pointed out, it takes time for the level to fall from a pre-diagnosis high. The mother initially did not see things that way, and the figure of 55 attached itself to the boy's body as if he were still sick. The nurse was able to nuance the mother's reading of the situation, spelling out that the figure should be taken as a positive sign and testimony to the parents' successful management of their son's diabetes at home.

The blood test complete, it was time to see the doctor. The nurse showed the family into the room where the doctor was waiting, and sat down on a chair. This marked it as a new situation, with the doctor leading the clinical encounter. She began by looking at the boy and asking 'Have you got any questions', but the boy said nothing. Instead, the mother said, 'You do have a question. How long do people have this disease?' The doctor looked at the boy and said, 'You have it all the time, but you're well. You have to take your medicine or you can get very sick'. The nurse filled in by saying 'Did you hear that?' Just as the nurse had initially visualized two bodies, one before and one after treatment began, the doctor's answer to the boy's question also actualized two bodies. If the parents were to successfully treat their son as prescribed, the health service would define him as having a healthy body, meaning almost life as normal before the diabetes diagnosis (Nilsson & Hansson 2016); fail in the treatment and diabetes would emerge again, and the boy would count as ill, which would be reflected in the HbA1c test.

After their opening exchange, the doctor addressed the parents directly to comment on the HbA1c test. Like the nurse earlier, she said 'It's looking good, it's on the right track.' She then explained

HbA1c. Both the doctor and the nurse used the same travel metaphor: the family would travel ahead in time and their hard work would be rewarded with better figures. Metaphors are common in healthcare, used to translate abstract reasoning into more manageable facts (Lakoff & Johnson 1980; Sontag 1989; Gustafsson & Hommerberg 2016). Here too there is another body—a body that is not static but changes over time, and for which parents must invest time and commitment if the HbA1c is to fall within the target values. It is standard for these metaphors to be framed as stories about the future; in the clinical encounter, this is about what the patient, or the family, can achieve if they follow medical advice. Medical advice often takes the form of *instrumental narratives*, focusing on the procedures involved in the treatment (Hansson 2007), as against the stories about the future, which are rather *moral narratives* about the state of health patients and families should aim for, focused on an imagined future in which the patient has improved, and frequently with an ethical dimension about the extent of patient or family responsibility for the disease and its treatment (Ricoeur 1990; Frid 2004). At the same time, in the clinical encounter there is an obligation on patients or families to accept these stories about the reasons for treatment (Hansson 2007).

One such instrumental narrative was the next stage in the consultation, when the doctor moved on from the HbA1c test to the blood sugar data which the family had uploaded with the nurse's help when they arrived at the clinic. When the doctor looked at the figures, shown as a curve on her computer screen, she had nothing but praise for the family's efforts to take responsibility for their son's treatment: 'He's following his curve perfectly; he's following it perfectly,' she said. Since the doctor was so positive, the consultation took another turn as the mother and the doctor went over the Social Insurance Agency paperwork which would allow the mother to be at home with her son a while longer. To bring the consultation to a close, the doctor turned to both parents and said 'Anything else that's happened?' The father now joined the conversation, saying 'There were some weird values where it shot up,' adding that the nurse had 'told us why, that is that he was going down with something'. The father continued, trying to give a medical explanation for why he thought the numbers odd. The doctor's response to this was not to answer directly, but to ask briefly 'What doses is he on?' The mother gave the insulin doses as a sequence of figures for a twenty-four-hour period. The doctor, looking for an answer, then wanted to know what his afternoon dose was. The mother turned to the father for help but he looked blank, so the mother got out her mobile phone, where she had all the doses noted down. After a little searching she found the value the doctor had asked for. The doctor brought up the day in question on her screen, and looking at it said 'That looks fine to me'. The nurse now joined in, pointing at the value and asking 'Was it that one?' to which the mother said yes, and the doctor once again pointed out 'He's not that low there. You get what we call recoil, because the body counteracts with hormones. Much later you get a higher value,' she added, pointing at the screen.

In this way, moral narratives also surfaced about the family's normal life—their lifeworld (Husserl 2002)—and how it related to the boy's figures. The parents had tried to come up with an answer for what the different figures meant. In the clinical encounter their lifeworld altered so it was now the physician, and partly the nurse, who had the interpretive precedence in explaining the figures. The doctor seemed unworried by the parents' anxiety. In this way, at least two further bodies took their place in the clinical encounter. There was the body the parents dealt with every day, seen when they tried to grasp what they felt was a variety of figures, and there was also a more medicalized body that the doctor could easily define as completely within the hoped-for normal values. The doctor was satisfied with how the parents had taken responsibility for the instrumental narrative—how best to manage the child's diabetes—and in that way had taken responsibility for the moral narrative too.

The mother, though, was not satisfied, and continued to discuss her thoughts about the boy's different figures with the doctor, giving different scenarios from their daily life and explaining her thinking. The doctor listened and gave her picture of things, while the father stayed out of the conversation. At one point, the mother said 'We talked it over' to make it clear she had her husband's support, but her 'we' was largely governed by her being the one at home with their son and shouldering much of the responsibility for his treatment. Thus, there also appeared to be two bodies in the family's daily life: the mother's view of the boy's body as one that had to be cared for; and the father stepping back and entrusting responsibility for the boy's body to the mother. This view of the boy's body was also evident in the father's comment that 'We're squabbling a fair bit' about what figures the boy should have. The doctor tried to help the parents agree, and said straightaway that the boy should be around 6 for a good HbA1c. 'What I said', said the mother, displaying that she was taking responsibility for the child's body. Towards the end of the consultation, the division became even clearer when it transpired that the mother had been worried by the boy's body and figures: she said that now 'I don't feel that kind of stress' about the figures, and the doctor praised her with the words 'That's good, important', while the father added, 'You've calmed down'. The mother's response was 'Thank you', to which the doctor said, 'It's a lot', referring to the burden carried by the mother on a daily basis.

With Mol's concept (2002) of the body multiple, we can see how one and the same body can be interpreted and understood in different situations, and that it affects—enacts—how each individual relates to the figures from that body. The figures are thus not only a form of standardized knowledge, circulating freely in the clinical encounter, but to a far greater extent they also have the character of things, shaping and shaped by the individuals who use that knowledge (Agamben 2014). These are the same figures that the doctor, nurse, mother, and father see, but they all seem to respond differently. Here, the worries voiced by the mother are perhaps most revealing about her adoption of a mothering role, where the figures—the dispositif—seem to speak to her concerns about their child's health and well-being (Agamben 2014). Blood sugar levels are now central to her lifeworld, but HbA1c was in a way proof of whether she had succeeded or not. HbA1c is not only a value that categorizes the child's body, it also recruits the mother into caring for that body. Measurements and standardization thus create not only standardized knowledge of the child's body in a variety of situations, but also the subjectification processes by which the mother evolves a specific form of self-care for the child's body, with HbA1c the ratification process that distinguishes this body from the rest as an autonomous object in the world, and simultaneously creates a desubjectification process whereby the mother is drawn into that specific form of self-care (Agamben 2014). The self-care the mother has to adhere to is of the medical professionals' making, and in the clinical encounter she does not get across her realities in her own lifeworld, whether to her husband or to the doctor.

The figure of 52 is expressed in various ways in the clinical encounter, being bound up with the medical narratives and practices that the parents relate to in their lifeworld (Kleinman 1988). A central perspective when critiquing how medical 'facts' become autonomous things, being dispositif in our daily lives, is Edmund Husserl's *Die Krisis der europäischen Wissenschaften und die transzendentale Phänomenologie* of 1936. He described 'psychologism' as a discipline that distorts the human subject within its own lifeworld; his was a critique of modernity and of how it generates the desubjectification processes that alienate, here, the patient and their relatives in their own lifeworlds.[8] There is no need to claim that the figure of 52 distorts the family in their lifeworld for us to use the perspective to identify the practices changed and renegotiated in the clinical encounter, where the medical perspective prevails at the expense of the family's personal experience. It should be recognized that standardized knowledge not only is generated in the clinical encounter, but has obvious power differentials there, and impacts how the family sees the doctor and the nurse.[9] Despite the criticism, as this particular consultation drew to a close the parents seemed satisfied. They had been given new information to take home, where they would continue caring for their son in the best manner possible.

The professionals and 52

To understand why the figure of 52 is so important in the clinical encounter, we must look beyond patients and families' needs for information in managing diabetes in their daily lives. The figure is also of great importance for how medical staff, and especially doctors and nurses, think and talk about what they do. As we have seen, HbA1c today is comparable not only individually, but also as a metric of all the diabetes clinics in the country, and thus a control mechanism—'know-how'—for relations between various clinics, between clinics and hospital management, between clinics and government, between clinics and patient associations, and so on (Rose & Miller 1992). As the literature has found, it presents the opportunity to manage a clinic from a distance, for example by defining the range of target values the clinic should meet (Latour 1987; Bloomfield 1991). Here 52 is little more than a control mechanism that determines hospital care by labelling specific forms of performance in the health service (Tøndel 2017).[10] A key point in this is found in the literary analyses by Knut Ove Eliassen (2008), who writes that naming—in the sense of designation—is not only about giving people individual identities that make it possible to follow them throughout their lives, but is also about identifying things. It is by naming that the world becomes understandable to an organization, while the organization is distanced from the world by the act of naming. Eliassen's point is similar to the subjectification and desubjectification processes already described, but here the focus is instead the organization (Nilsson & Sjöstedt Landén 2017).

The question of HbA1c arose at the first staff meeting I observed. Although the meeting was about something else, they still ended up discussing the figure of 52 and whether the clinic should work to have the best average value in Sweden, which was not then the case. The doctor who was head of the clinic said that 'We're going to be the best team in Sweden', and that they should work to allow patients to become independent, supported with the correct knowledge to manage their diabetes. The fact that the lead doctor could even suggest it was because the clinic had joined a network of diabetes clinics across Sweden, where each submitted their HbA1c averages and thus made themselves comparable—a control mechanism for the clinics, as the figures determine a number of their priorities. Also, however, this had given rise to certain idioms. Some of the medical staff had attended a national conference where various clinics' averages had been compared, and at a staff meeting on their return said 'It's fun that the HbA1c has gone down', while another interjected 'It's nice, it takes a while to see the change'.

To achieve this goal, the endocrinology department would have to be unequivocal with families and patients about the blood sugar levels they were to aim for. At the staff meeting, one nurse responsible for the HbA1c work said that the clinic 'should continue working on high HbA1c', supporting families who have not got their child's diabetes treatment under control. One way was to be clear with families and give them the leaflet discussed at the start of this chapter, as it spells out the guidelines the clinic expects families to follow in daily life. One of the doctors said how important it was to 'show the document to those who are going over 60', indicating it was crucial to identify the patients who needed extra help. The figure of 52 was thus not only a control mechanism that shaped the clinic's operations, but also served as a marker for those patients who failed to meet the target.

It was imperative that staff identify and engage with families and patients who fell outside the target values, as their health was at risk of deterioration and they needed extra support in their self-care, and they pushed up the clinic's average HbA1c. One late afternoon, shortly after one of the staff meetings I observed, I was walking with some of the doctors and nurses through the hospital. They were chatting a little more freely as it was not a formal meeting, and the conversation turned to the clinic's 'duffers', who had poor HbA1c values and glucometer readings that were all over the place, and who doctors felt were not telling staff the truth about how they managed their diabetes. In informal conversation, these patients became actors who not only risked their own health, but also ensured the clinic had worse results than the other clinics in Sweden. One of the staff said that it only took a single patient like that to affect the clinic's national ranking.[11]

The healthcare professionals kept coming back to this form of categorization, worrying about how to get medical information across to patients and families. There was one such dialogue at a staff meeting about coming to grips with patients who failed to meet the guidelines set by the endocrinology department. One of the doctors noted that one particular family was finding things exceedingly difficult, because the father had diabetes too and never checked his blood sugar and the mother had cancer. Their son's blood sugar levels were worrying, and the doctor asked 'Who is going to support this boy?' The doctor's suggestion was to try a home visit. Another of the doctors, picking up on the idea, said 'I think you're absolutely right, we have to find new ways. But at the same time, hospital appointments are important for getting things to work.' The first doctor's response was that 'For some it feels utterly pointless. This is a patient who needs help making treatment part of normal life.' One of the nurses said home visits that should not be routine, but could be an important 'tool in the toolbox'. A third doctor suggested 'finding an ally at the school', but the nurses pointed out that it needed considerable effort to make that work. The doctor who sparked the discussion ended it by saying 'Those with a high HbA1c are the ones we haven't reached; if we had, we wouldn't have them.'

In the discussions between the medical staff the notion of an ideal family can be glimpsed—one that has developed its self-care, and with it not only an understanding of the diabetic child's body, but also of how the family can take responsibility for the diabetes treatment. Yet there are also those who fall outside this, where neither the family nor the child seems able to take responsibility as the medical staff wish they would: they lack what in healthcare is known as compliance (Arduser 2017). It is as if these bodies defy the clinic's ways of categorizing and organizing patients, and are instead identified as anomalies that must be persuaded back into the system one way or another. Many of the meetings I observed were about how doctors, nurses, dieticians, or counsellors could best talk to these patients and families: how to teach them and how to reach out to them in their lifeworlds. Central to this was individualized care, tailored to meet the needs of the individual or family 'where they are', and at the same time give them the tools to make their own decisions—but it was obvious that not all families were anywhere near that. As for the more problematic patients—the 'duffers'—staff could report them to social services as a final recourse. As one of the doctors said at a staff meeting, she 'doesn't report the ones who are finding it hard going as long as they're not stroppy', but at the same time she wondered aloud, 'How long can they be up at 110?' None of those present ventured to answer, but all understood the trouble with such a high figure when the goal was for everyone to be 52 or below.

What my ethnographic cultural analysis shows is there is a form of enactment, as Mol (2002) points out, which is influenced by the tools the staff can enact with. There are no predetermined subjects, for they are created by the healthcare practices, whether a staff meeting or a clinical encounter. Here Mol, invoking Judith Butler in *Gender Trouble* (1990), notes that the subject 'is not given but practiced. The pervasive and mundane acts in which this is done make people what they are' (2002, 37). HbA1c is just such a tool in the medical practices where the body multiple is defined and categorized as a form of enactment, and thus appears as normal and unproblematic—or as an anomaly that the healthcare system must work particularly hard to bring back into the medical fold. Central to Mol's theory (2002) is her argument that medicine is nothing if not an exercise in power, where the strongest form of enactment is the one that can be imposed. In this she is informed by Bruno Latour's dictum that 'The strongest reason always yields to the reason of the strongest' (Latour 1993, cited in Mol 2002, 108). The strongest reason identified here would appear to be the figures—the dispositifs (Agamben 2014)—for HbA1c, and their power to categorize bodies according to practice, and thus to enter the lifeworlds of patients and families, affecting their relationship with the treatment and a normal life with diabetes. This form of categorization seems based on the healthcare system's requirements, though, and not necessarily the patients' or the families' best interests, despite the patient's best interest being the first thing any healthcare professional would point to as the reason it is so important to track HbA1c and blood sugar levels. The standardized knowledge associated with the figure of 52 directly affects how bodies—in this chapter seen as bodies multiple—are categorized and related to in different practices.

Conclusions

The figure of 52 is found in this chapter to be a thing, a dispositif, which exerts a centripetal force on a range of practices in Swedish diabetes care and beyond. It is not only a figure for patients and families to aim for in managing the disease, it also generates a relationship of sorts between them and medical staff, *and* it affects healthcare provision and how staff design patient care and categorize patients. The result is that 52 is an ethnographic route to understanding how today's medicine objectifies, measures, and standardizes the diabetes care on offer. In the chapter, this is discussed in terms of subjectification and desubjectification processes, where patients, families, and staff are all subject to the HbA1c test's ordering of reality (Agamben 2014). While the figure engenders practices which the actors should enact in their everyday lives—at home or in hospital—it simultaneously renders other practices impossible.

Central here is the fact that the figure of 52 can be considered standardized knowledge. This form of knowledge is not necessarily mutable or even mouldable; rather, it is locked into a specific state of knowing about what diabetes is and how it should be best treated. Standardization makes it awkward for patients, families, and staff to question the figure, and so it continues as a point of reference, as something to comment on or relate to. HbA1c not only generates and controls a number of practices, but those practices are self-sustaining and can be said to underscore the significance of the figure of 52 in diabetes care. Given the way HbA1c has been used, its standardizing function is fixed, confirming it as the key perspective in healthcare of this type.

Diabetes care is just one of many examples of healthcare where we can see a similar trend, with figures being increasingly central to standardized knowledge processes of all kinds. To some extent, this development has been driven by new control mechanisms in healthcare and digitalization. Today's healthcare control mechanisms are designed to turn healthcare practices not only into categorizable figures, but also into figures that can be followed up and compared; and different strategies can be chosen according to how the figures are categorized (Pollitt & Bouckaert 2000). It is in its figures the organization manifests itself and thus exercises a degree of control over its operations (Bornemark 2018). But it is not only in relation to its organization that figures have become increasingly central to the health service; in the form of quality registry data, figures are essential in shaping views of specific diagnoses or whether a treatment should be retained or altered (Lindh & Rivano Eckerdal 2016). Ongoing digitalization has made it easier to compile large quantities of data and compare them by patient, by clinic, or by region. Without digitalization, it is hard to imagine that this particular standardized knowledge could have expanded as it did. Many patients' HbA1c readings, combined with other facts and figures over prolonged periods makes it possible to compare, develop, and change healthcare.

The significance of 52 thus stems from the practices in which it operates, and with the help of Mol's perspective (2002) we can discuss the body multiple and its interpretations, which vary from practice to practice. The concept of the body multiple is an indication of how standardized knowledge is coded and embedded in a context with multiple exclusion mechanisms (Foucault 1993), where some perspectives are defined as problematic or are rendered invisible, while others are categorized as important. This dispositif offers actors the prospect of action while eliminating other activities, so that actors are subjected to the way HBA1c—or the figure of 52—arranges reality.

The purpose of this chapter has been to examine how figures can create normative guidelines in a medical setting, and how they are interpreted and used according to their contextual practices, setting out in brief what these normative guidelines might mean. However, as is evident from the ethnography, there is also the crucial factor that standardized knowledge does not in any way, shape, or form standardize the lived lifeworlds of patients, families, and staff. Rather, the figure of 52 is something to relate to, for it is only then the figure is set in motion, knowledge and all.

Notes

1 In Sweden, where the study was conducted, the public health service is the responsibility of 21 health regions. There are thus variations in organization and supply, but in most regions all non-hospital care is free for children and adolescents under the age of 20. Prescription medicines are free for those under the age 18, as are most medical aids.

2 The target value was subsequently reduced and at time of writing is 48 mmol/mol.

3 The HbA1c test requires expensive equipment—not something a family can have at home, although they can take blood samples at home and send them in to a pathology laboratory. In most Swedish hospitals the HbA1c test machine is in the diabetes clinic, where it is convenient for patients to be tested during regular appointments.

4 The leaflet is above all a document (Buckland 1997, see Markus Idvall's chapter in this book)—and an element in the dispositif—which can create a variety of values for families. To be handed the document can be the closing ritual of a clinical encounter (Whyte et al. 2002); it might be thought a gift of trust which the family now has to take responsibility for (Mauss 2001); it can be a non-human actor linking the family's actions with the health service (Latour 1992). In my thesis (Hansson 2007), I write about another class of medical document with similar characteristics: prescriptions. A prescription too can act as a closing ritual, leaving the patient at the end of a consultation feeling positive about their medical problems (Whyte et al. 2002, 123 ff.), and in the position to actualize their treatment with their own personal medical object. But like any medical object, a prescription also refers to the doctor and their instructions, 'freezing' the spoken word as writing or thing, which only enhances the doctor's authority.

5 Gabriella Nilsson and I have drawn attention to this elsewhere, arguing that its effect is to encourage families to alter their view of their child's diabetes from a disease perspective to a lifestyle perspective, where the disease, rather than a limit on life, is seen as part of life (Nilsson & Hansson 2016, 262).

6 A lifeworld is also commonly equated with morphological structure, for even though

it is an inaccurate, intersubjective consciousness, the lifeworld still builds on scientific knowledge or countenances scientific knowledge (Wallenstein 2011).

7 This is a form of desubjectification: it is virtually impossible for the family and the patient to avoid the dispositif, and instead they are subject to HbA1c's specific way of ordering reality (Agamben 2014). As per Martin Heidegger (2013), this process is a form of alienation that modern people can extricate themselves from only with difficulty.

8 Alienation is the term Karl Marx (2018) coined for his critical theory of modernity, and it can also be found in Husserl (1993), albeit with a slightly different meaning. In this chapter, it is applied to the dispositif, and with it the web of power which envelopes the individual, but which may be difficult to see or criticize (Agamben 2014; see also Heidegger 2013). These systems of power can be capitalist—Marx—or scientific—Husserl.

9 In this I follow Michel Foucault's argument (2003) that power creates counter-power, but it is for another occasion to explore what patients and families can do in the face of these power structures.

10 This is comparable to the umbrella term of new public management, which describes how public services mimic business organizations, for example by defining metrics as targets to be followed up and evaluated (Pollitt & Bouckaert 2000; Karlsson 2017).

11 Not that staff could not provide excellent care for their patients otherwise—during my fieldwork, for example, I heard of a doctor who had his mobile phone on outside working hours so patients and families could ring for help in managing daily life—but rather it marks a form of (de)subjectification process, by which healthcare professionals subjectify individuals and take extra care of them, while desubjectifying them by translating them into figures and values to be managed.

References

Agamben, Giorgio (2014), *Vad är ett dispositiv?* (Malmö: Eskaton).

Alftberg, Åsa & Kristofer Hansson (2012), 'Introduction: Self-care translated into practice', *Culture Unbound: Journal of Current Cultural Research*, 4, 415–24.

Arduser, Lora (2017), *Living chronic: Agency and expertise in the rhetoric of diabetes* (Columbus: Ohio State University Press).

Beckman, Anita (2009), *Väntan: Etnografiskt kollage kring ett mellanrum* (Gothenburg: Mara).

Bloomfield, Brian P. (1991), 'The role of information systems in the UK national health service: Action at a distance and the fetish of calculation', *Social Studies of Science*, 21(4), 701–734.

Bornemark, Jonna (2018), *Det omätbaras renässans: En uppgörelse med pedanternas världsherravälde* (Stockholm: Volante).

Buckland, Michael K. (1997), 'What is a "document"?', *Journal of the American Society for Information Science*, 48(9), 804–809.

Butler, Judith (1990), *Gender trouble: Feminism and the subversion of identity* (New York: Routledge).

Ehn, Billy & Orvar Löfgren (2010), *The secret world of doing nothing* (Berkeley & Los Angeles: University of California Press).

Eliassen, Knut Ove (2008), 'Tingens tale: Epistemologi, estetikk og eksistens hos Michel Foucault', *Norsk filosofisk tidskrift*, 43(4), 290–303.

Fioretos, Ingrid, Kristofer Hansson & Gabriella Nilsson (2013), *Vårdmöten: Kulturanalytiska perspektiv på möten inom vården* (Lund: Studentlitteratur).

Foucault, Michel (1978), *Histoire de la sexualité*, i: *La volonté de savoir* (Paris: Gallimard).

—— (1993), *Diskursens ordning: Installationsföreläsning vid Collège de France den 2 december 1970* (Stockholm: Brutus Östlings Bokförlag Symposion).

—— (2003), Övervakning och straff: Fängelsets födelse (4th rev. edn, Lund: Arkiv).

Frid, Ingvar (2004), 'Att ta del av en berättelse: En resa mot okänt mål', in Carola Skott (ed.), *Berättelsens praktik och teori: Narrativ forskning i ett hermeneutiskt perspektiv* (Lund: Studentlitteratur).

Frykman, Jonas & Nils Gilje (2003), 'Being there: An introduction', in eid. (eds.), *Being there: New perspectives on phenomenology and the analysis of culture* (Lund: Nordic Academic Press).

Gadamer, Hans-Georg (1996). *The enigma of health: The art of healing in a scientific age.* Cambridge: Polity Press.

Gustafsson, Anna W. & Charlotte Hommerberg (2016), '"Pojken lyfter sitt svärd: Ger sig in i en strid han inte kan vinna": Om metaforer och kronisk cancersjukdom', *Socialmedicinsk tidskrift*, 93(3), 271–279.

Hacking, Ian (1999), *The social construction of what?* (Cambridge, MA: Harvard University Press).

Hansson, Kristofer (2007), *I ett andetag: En kulturanalys av astma som begränsning och möjlighet* (Stockholm: Critical Ethnography Press).

—— (2013), 'En mångfaldig forskningsetik', *Rig*, 164–70.

Heidegger, Martin (2013[1927]), *Vara och tid* (Gothenburg: Daidalos).

Husserl, Edmund (1993 [1936]), *Husserliana: Gesammelte Werke*, xxix: *Die Krisis der Europäischen Wissenschaften und die transzendentale Phänomenologie, Ergänzungsband, Texte aus dem Nachlass 1934–1937* (Dordrecht: Kluwer).

—— (2002 [1913]), *Husserliana: Gesammelte Werke*, xx/1: *Logische Untersuchungen: Ergänzungsband: Entwürfe zur Umarbeitung der VI. Untersuchung und zur Vorrede für die Neuauflage der Logischen Untersuchungen* (Dordrecht: Kluwer).

Karlsson, Tom S. (2017), *New public management: Ett nyliberalt 90-talsfenomen?* (Lund: Studentlitteratur).

Kleinman, Arthur (1988), *The illness narratives: Suffering, healing, and the human condition* (New York: Basic).

Lakoff, George & Mark Johnson (1980), *Metaphors we live by* (Chicago: University of Chicago Press).

Larsen, Tord & Emil A. Røyrvik (2017), introduction to eid. (eds.), *Trangen til å telle: Objektivering, måling og standardisering som samfunnspraksis* (Oslo: Scandinavian Adademic Press).

Latour, Bruno (1987), *Science in action: How to follow scientists and engineers through society* (Cambridge, MA: Harvard University Press).

—— (1992/1998), 'Teknik är samhället som gjorts hållbart', in id., *Artefaktens återkomst: Ett möte mellan organisationsteori och tingens sociologi* (Stockholm: Nerenius & Santérus).

—— Alan Sheridan & John Law (1993 [1988]), *The pasteurization of France* (Cambridge, MA: Harvard University Press).

Lindh, Karolina & Johanna Rivano Eckerdal (2016), 'Livsdugliga data i gränslandet mellan vård, styrdokument och teknik', *Socialmedicinsk tidskrift*, 93(3), 297–305.

Marcus, George E. (1995), 'Ethnography in/of the world system: The emergence of multi-sited ethnography', *Annual Reviews of Anthropology*, 24.

Marx, Karl (2018 [1867]), *Kapitalet, i: Kapitalets produktionsprocess* (7th edn, Lund: Arkiv förlag/A-Z förlag).

Mauss, Marcel (2001 [1902]), *A general theory of magic* (London: Routledge Classics).

Mol, Annemarie (2002), *The body multiple: Ontology in medical practice* (Durham: Duke University Press).

Nilsson, Gabriella & Angelika Sjöstedt Landén (2017), 'Arbetslivsetnologi: Professioner i nyliberala organisationer', *Kulturella perspektiv: Svensk etnologisk tidsskrift*, 26, 2–7.

Nilsson, Gabriella & Kristofer Hansson (2016), 'Berättade fantasier om förr, nu och framtiden i vården av barn med diabetes', *Socialmedicinsk tidskrift*, 93(3), 261–270.

Pollitt, Christopher & Geert Bouckaert (2000) *Public management reform* (Oxford: OUP).

Prout, Alan (1996), 'Actor–network theory, technology and medical sociology: An illustrative analysis of the metered dose inhaler', *Sociology of Health & Illness*, 18(2), 198–219.

Ricoeur, Paul (1990/1994), *Oneself as another* (Chicago: University of Chicago Press).

Rose, Nicolas & Peter Miller (1992), 'Political power beyond the state: Problematics of government', *British Journal of Sociology*, 43(2), 173–205.

Skott, Carola (2013) (ed.), *Människan i vården: Etnografi, vård och drama* (Stockholm: Carlsson).

Sontag, Susan (1989), *Illness as metaphor and AIDS and its metaphors* (New York: Picador/Farrar, Straus & Giroux).

Tøndel, Gunhild (2017), 'Omsorgens håndtrykk i scener rundt tall', in Tord Larsen & Emil A. Røyrvik (eds.), *Trangen til å telle: Objektivering, måling og standardisering som samfunnspraksis* (Oslo: Scandinavian Adademic Press).

Wallenstein, Sven-Olov (2011), 'Husserl, tekniken och livsvärlden', *Fenomenologi, teknik & medialitet*, 21–54.

Whyte, Susan Reynolds, Sjaak van der Geest & Anita Hardon (2002), *Social lives of medicines.* (Cambridge: Cambridge University Press).

CHAPTER 8

Knowledge worlds apart

Aesthetic experience as an epistemological boundary object

Max Liljefors

In November 2019, the World Health Organization (WHO) released one of its evidence reports, which it had commissioned on the positive health effects of the arts, *What is the evidence on the role of the arts in improving health and well-being*? (Fancourt & Finn 2019). It is far from the first to show that doing and experiencing art can have healing and rehabilitative effects, but the WHO report is the most comprehensive of its kind to date.[1] With its global perspective (albeit with an emphasis on Europe), it brings together findings from nearly 4,000 scholarly studies. Art's effects are found to span the entire human life cycle, from antenatal to geriatric and palliative care, and to take many forms, whether faster rehabilitation, reduced medication, fewer doctor's visits, the alleviation of a variety of physical and mental symptoms, and greater well-being and quality of life. The report concludes that the arts can have both health and socio-economic benefits, and should therefore be integrated into the WHO's European health policy, Health 2020.[2]

The WHO's evidence report is the most ambitious to date, with far-reaching ramifications for art and health as a field of research. In terms of the humanities, however, the most startling thing about the report is the knowledge that is not there, the knowledge that is noticeable by its absence. The report lacks any reference to the aesthetic disciplines—art history, musicology, literary studies, theatre studies—which traditionally steward the academic legacy of arts scholarship and continue to push back the boundaries. When the WHO report enumerates the theoretical basis of the studies it includes—'psychology, psychiatry, epidemiology, philosophy, ecology, history, health economics, neuroscience, medicine, health geography, public health, anthropology, and sociology, among others' (Fancourt & Finn 2019, 52)—there is not a word about the aesthetic disciplines. At best, their inclusion is implied by 'history', 'philosophy', or 'others'. The WHO report is not unique in this. In the field of arts and health, aesthetic subjects are significantly under-represented compared to medicine and healthcare.

It is only in recent decades that arts and health came together as a unified, international field of research. How did it come about that the aesthetic subjects, with learned traditions that date back centuries, have such a small part to play? It is no exaggeration to say that two worlds of knowledge have formed around art and the experience of art—two epistemological fields with the same object of study, which for simplicity's sake I refer to as the 'aesthetic experience', but which by and large are untroubled by academic exchange with each other.[3] One world of knowledge consists of the aesthetic disciplines as pursued in the humanities, the other of the various branches of scholarship in the field of arts and health. Why do they talk to each other so little? Could they, should they communicate more?

One object of study, separate worlds of knowledge

The prevailing situation means that the aesthetic experience has evolved into an epistemological boundary object. The concept of boundary objects was introduced by Susan Leigh Star and James R. Griesemer (1989) as a term for things and information that have a variety of meanings, and are handled in different ways in different social contexts, but which nevertheless have a settled content that ensures they are delimited in the same fashion, whatever the context. As a concept, it has gained currency in the theorization of interdisciplinary research. Writing on 'Credibility and Legitimacy' (2012), Elin Bommenel considers how it is that boundary objects facilitate communication between different branches of scholarship. When a variety of disciplines study the same object, it is usually with differing views of knowledge. Each discipline has its own research questions, methods, and results, which are considered legitimate and worthwhile. These knowledge criteria, Bommenel explains, have a dual function, for they guarantee scholarly quality within each discipline, while serving as a mechanism to exclude representatives of other academic (and non-academic) traditions. Interdisciplinary research into boundary objects requires researchers to lift their eyes from their own particular specialisms in two ways. The first is to accept that other disciplines operate under the principles of other knowledge criteria that are just as valid as their own criteria in their own field. The second (which is closely linked to the first) is to view their own criteria from a meta perspective as just one of several paths to knowledge. To have one's horizons broadened in this way is not to lessen the scholarly relevance of one's own knowledge criteria. What it does do, however, is encourage researchers to see whether lessons learnt from other disciplines can enrich their own fields, and whether their own knowledge has perhaps unanticipated relevance to other disciplines.

In what follows, I will discuss what is arguably a key factor in the different views of knowledge between the humanities' aesthetic studies and arts and health: the question of the instrumentalization of art. I also have a tentative proposal for how to bridge the epistemological gap, at least provisionally. A central role is played by the 'co-production of knowledge', a concept coined by Sheila Jasanoff (2004a, 3) to describe how knowledge is both the result of various scholarly disciplines' systematic studies of reality *and* various social and political interests. Co-production, as Jasanoff points out, is not a theory that claims comprehensive explanatory validity, but rather should be seen as an idiom, an interpretive perspective with which to avoid falling into the traps of social or scientific determinism, by recognizing both nature and society as factors in knowledge production (Jasanoff 2004a, 3; Jasanoff 2004b, 20). An interpretative, negotiating idiom of this type is particularly useful in interdisciplinary research about epistemological boundary objects, as it is neutral on the question of the hierarchy of different forms of knowledge. As she puts it:

> Unlike 'laws of nature', the idiom of co-production does not seek to foreclose competing explanations by laying claim to one dominant and all-powerful truth. It offers instead a new way of exploring the waters of human history, where politics, knowledge, and invention are continually in flux. (Jasanoff 2004b, 43)

Like Markus Idvall in his analysis of informed consent in the present volume, I draw inspiration from an article by Vololona Rabeharisoa and Michel Callon (2004) about how laypeople—patients and relatives—have successfully contributed to advances in French biomedical research on muscular dystrophy. Rabeharisoa and Callon apply the co-production perspective to the interaction between laypeople and experts. I will do something similar here, but first I consider the exchange of knowledge between experts in different fields. The differences are smaller than might at first appear: an expert in one discipline is usually a layperson in most other disciplines. It is Rabeharisoa and Callon's concept of 'intermediary discourse' that has immediate bearing on my argument. They use the term for a two-way discourse between experts and laypeople, a form of communication that is deliberately held at a level that is neither exclusively technical nor strategic, and designed so that laypeople (remembering that in interdisciplinary research everyone is a layperson to some extent) can gain an insight into the research process without being swamped by technicalities. According to Rabeharisoa and Callon, it is about 'going into the content of research without getting lost in it, that is to say, without losing sight of the goals' (151).

Their use of the word 'goal' indicates that the research they have studied had a clear purpose, as in addition to the usual vague scholarly ambition of increasing the sum of human knowledge their aim was to alleviate or cure a specific disease. This has direct relevance to my case here, since the gap that I argue exists between the aesthetic disciplines and the field of arts and health only exists courtesy of the instrumentalization of art—that is, whether the aesthetic experience can and should be anything other than an end in itself. The question of ends and means is also interesting because Bommenel (2012, 282) stipulates that successful interdisciplinary research demands that researchers from various disciplines agree on a common vision for their research goals. I believe this should be nuanced somewhat, since research is often conducted with several goals in mind, each with different degrees of generality, and specific goals do not necessarily have to be covered by the more general ones. I will return to the question of research objectives later.

The question of instrumentalization

The aesthetic disciplines command a wide repertoire of theoretical frameworks and analytical methods, which fall outside the scope of this study. The same is true of arts and health, if not even more so, because the field brings together so many disciplines. Aesthetic experiences are subjective in nature, and it is not obvious how their effects should be measured. As a rule, the medical and health sciences work with randomized controlled trials, quantitative designs, and predefined health outcomes, while ethnological research uses small case studies, qualitative analyses, and a strong element of argument and interpretation (Priebe & Sager 2014, 69–70). The result is very different types of data, so their mutual weighting is not straightforward. Studies tend to avoid talking in terms of cause and effect, and instead look for 'correlations' between art and health. A British report calls for a 'realistic approach', to include verifiable data of several kinds (APPGAHW 2017, 40–2). The WHO Evidence Report also holds back from specifying a hierarchy of different types of data and methods.

Given such a diverse field of research, it may seem surprising that the aesthetic disciplines do not already play a prominent part, especially as they have several centuries' head start on the systematic study of the arts. The reason why, I believe, is not so much specific methods and theories, and more the underlying approach to the object of study, art. Kristofer Hansson and Rachel Irwin make the point in the introduction to this volume that value judgements about the validity of different forms of knowledge determine the direction taken by clinical research. This is no less true of aesthetics. In the history of art—I focus on my own discipline, Art History, in the belief that scholars in other aesthetic subjects can identify with my arguments—there is a firm conviction that art should not be subject to the requirement of being useful, that it should not be instrumentalized. Art scholars leap to the defence of the freedom of art whenever politicians set about controlling public art or the Church censors 'inappropriate' artworks. This is not only a political response, but stems from profound epistemological perspectives. It is worth dwelling on the most important.

The discipline of art history is strongly influenced by aesthetic philosophy, which periodically has been closely intertwined with art theory. The view that the aesthetic experience is essentially different to other types of experience is particularly dominant. Immanuel Kant (1724–1804), in his magisterial third critique, *Critique of the Power of Judgment* (2002 [1790]), dissects the meaning of aesthetic judgement using a series of distinctions. The power of judgement constitutes its own form of knowledge, dissimilar to knowledge derived from pure reason and practical reason (the subjects of Kant's two previous critiques). He separates judgement into aesthetic and teleological judgement, of which the former exists as four different types. One of these is the judgement of beauty, which for Kant falls into 'adherent' beauty, which means that it is conditioned by an idea of the object having a purpose, or 'free' beauty, free from every notion of how the object should look or function. Only free beauty, according to Kant, can give rise to 'pure' aesthetic judgement, uncontaminated by instrumental considerations, and it is this form that is associated with the fine arts. Kant admits that aesthetic judgement in reality often exists in combination with other forms of judgement, and his third critique is indeed still subject to philosophical exegesis, but the point here is that art history has inherited the intellectual impulse to think about aesthetic experience in its purest form. It is primarily thought of in contrast to, and not together with, other forms of experience and receptiveness.

Other outlooks on knowledge are closely linked to this approach. Thus, history of art is traditionally noted for its analytical focus on the artwork per se, and the internal dynamics which give the artwork its distinct meaning-making and aesthetic force. Sweeping generalizations about different types of artworks or their historical origins are considered superficial, a sign of sloppy thinking. In short, each artwork should be presumed to constitute its own world of meanings—these can certainly vary in nature, depending on the historical context, but always manifest in and through the artwork itself.

Further, the discipline is wedded to a strong historiographical narrative that holds the (Western) history of art to be a progression towards independence and self-knowledge. In this view, art ever since the Enlightenment has gradually shed its political and religious shackles in order to focus on its own problems and an exploration of its own nature. Clement Greenberg (1982 [1965]), inspired by Kant, formulated one variation of this notion of history; Arthur Danto another (1997), in his case based on Friedrich Hegel's (1770–1831) philosophy of history.

I would not claim that all art historians today agree with the views outlined above—views which within the discipline have been subject to close, extended critiques—but, regardless, I would argue they are cornerstones of art history, and have done much to shape the knowledge criteria and values of the discipline. These criteria and values remain powerful, even when the underlying philosophical arguments retreat into the background or are abandoned. One such value is art history's deep scepticism about the instrumentalization of art. I believe this stems not so much from an impulse to defend artistic freedom, as a feeling that instrumentalization runs counter to the very definition of art, and, above all, challenges the basis of the discipline's knowledge criteria.

While utilitarianism in art is anathema to art history, the situation in arts and health is the opposite: art's usefulness in the shape of its positive health effects is the field's *raison d'être*. The knowledge criteria this gives rise to are very different. First, it is not the artwork itself that is the primary object of study, but the activities associated with the artwork—for example, a group of patients who discuss an exhibition they have seen, or who attend a creative workshop. The specifics of the artwork, its particularities and dynamics, rarely feature much in the analysis. Instead, the focus is the patients' physiological or psychological responses. Also, observable health effects in specific art activities are normally seen as the result of several interrelated factors. The aesthetic element coexists with other factors such as social interaction (activities often take place in groups) or physical movement, whose effects can rarely be isolated from one another. Moreover, health effects can be measured as physiological responses, such as stress hormone levels or cardiovascular reactivity, or as certain types of neuronal activity in the brain. This necessitates studies of variations on a physiological basis that is common to all mental states and processes. Arts and health, unlike the aesthetic disciplines, rarely pauses to consider the aesthetic experience in its pure, idealized form.

These disparities in knowledge criteria result in different types of statements. Art history's nuanced analyses seem to be of little relevance to arts and health, as they do not speak to that field's main concern, the effect of art on patients. For arts and health, the principle that art is possessed of categorical autonomy, separate from people's encounters with it, lacks epistemological value. Conversely, for art history, the references in arts and health to patients' observable responses are at best a trivialization of art. For art's worth to be dictated by such utilitarian externalities would be to instrumentalize it, to superficialize it in a manner that skids over the depths of meaning and meaningfulness that are intrinsic to the specificities of the work. Ultimately, statements made in the one sphere of knowledge do not meet the basic criteria for legitimate scholarship in the other.

There are exceptions, just as there are hybrid forms, and researchers in their respective spheres of knowledge are not unaware of one another's rationales and motives; however, the dividing lines are still so entrenched that knowledge exchanges between the fields are complicated, and thus far have been remarkably rare. How to make it easier? As an epistemological boundary object, can the aesthetic experience facilitate a reflective cross-disciplinary dialogue? As already noted, co-production is a fruitful way to think about knowledge, as it requires us to explicitly refrain from ranking the various forms of knowledge, the better to understand their inherent complexities. What, then, would be the contours of an 'intermediary discourse', as Rabeharisoa and Callon (2004) call it, which can bring together experts and laypeople (or experts from a variety of fields)? It is not a question of ignoring the differences in order to plough ahead and unify the criteria from all spheres of knowledge into a single coherent system. Rather, efforts should concentrate on identifying specific, local overlaps, preferably where the dividing lines are at their clearest. The instrumentalization of art offers just one such opportunity.

Existential health as the basis
for an intermediary discourse

To bridge the gap between the aesthetic disciplines and arts and health, one possibility is to reflect on the concept of health. When the WHO was founded in 1948, it adopted a three-pronged definition of health as 'a state of complete physical, mental and social well-being and not merely the absence of disease or infirmity'.[4] This has been criticized for being unrealistic, since no one is likely to achieve *complete* well-being in all three health dimensions, physical, mental, and social. But there have been calls from some quarters in recent years for the WHO's definition to be extended by the addition of another health dimension, usually referred to as *existential* or *spiritual health* (Sigurdson 2014; Melder 2011). The point of this fourth dimension would be to transect the other three, rather than being some sort of appendage. It is important to note that the term spiritual does not equate to religious, in the sense of confessional affiliation; rather, existential or spiritual health is about a subjective sense of meaningfulness, participation in something greater, and self-understanding. Insoo Hyun (2016, 128), who has studied spiritual distress in the face of illness, sees spirituality as the 'experiential and emotional aspects of personal connection, inner peace, and support', which some people find in religious traditions and others in nature, music, the arts or social community. Ola Sigurdson (2014, 34–6) distinguishes between spiritual and existential health, arguing that the existential dimension is characterized by self-reflection, which means that it cuts through or embraces all the other dimensions. That is the sense in which I use the term existential health here.

Atul Gawande's book *Being Mortal* (2014), about palliative care, provides some very useful insights. Gawande does not refer to existential health per se, but he writes about a form of well-being that captures much of what the concept is about. He believes that all care should reflect the fact that people are mortal. Accept that, he says, and care becomes more than a fight to extend the patient's life as long as possible. An equally important goal is to make it possible for the patient to experience meaningfulness and satisfaction, even when life is marked by illness, loss, or approaching death. Gawande uses the example of a study at Massachusetts General Hospital of a group of lung cancer patients who chose to combine standard oncology treatment with palliative care, where they were given support in thinking through what they found meaningful in life given their circumstances. When the researchers compared them with a control group who had chosen only the oncology treatment, those who had palliative care were found to experience a significantly higher quality of life and to exhibit fewer signs of depression. Further, the hospice group lived on average 25 per cent longer, despite receiving less life-sustaining treatment in the final stages of their illness (Gawande 2014, 177–8; see also Temel et al. 2010).

Gawande identifies two factors as crucial to this kind of well-being, which I argue is existential health in all but name. One is autonomy; the other is breaking the isolation that often accompanies illness. By autonomy, he does not mean an absence of external constraints—the freedom to do whatever you want—for it is obvious that life will be limited by illness and disability. Instead, it is an inner autonomy; the ability to experience meaningfulness even when your external life is much curtailed, and to find a way to relate to your life. In Gawande's words, it is about making space to be 'the authors of our lives', even in situations not of our choosing such as illness or imminent death (140). Such existential well-being may certainly come with objectively measurable health effects, as in the Massachusetts study, but it cannot be reduced to metrics or evaluated solely on the basis of quantifiable outcomes. Instead, it has intrinsic worth.

Existential health, if understood as inner autonomy and connection, shares a great deal with the characterization of aesthetic experience in the aesthetic disciplines. Therein lies its potential to bridge the gap, if only provisionally, between the two spheres of knowledge when it comes to the instrumentalization of art. This much is evident if we take a closer look at how certain philosophers have described the aesthetic experience. Since Kant, a key theme in aesthetic philosophy is the special kind of freedom that characterizes the aesthetic. Freedom from instrumental concerns gives free rein to both perception and cognition. Their free movement, a kind of inner play which is satisfying in itself, is shaped by a dual dynamic, which coincides well with Gawande's two aspects. On the one hand, the aesthetic creates a distance from mundane consciousness, leading to self-reflection; on the other, it gives an immediacy to the object viewed, and with that a greater sense of presence and participation (see Liljefors & Alftberg 2019).

Martin Seel (2014), pondering Hegel, Kant, and Adorno, talks of people's receptiveness to the aesthetic as an 'active passivity', a conscious willingness to accept experiences but never to grasp after them, to be unconditionally open to the dynamics of the artwork and its effects; an activity that involves being alert to aspects that mundane consciousness tends to overlook, a 'being-there-with and going-along-with an abundance of forms and relations that we usually fail to recognize in our everyday modes of relating to the world' (271). For Seel, an individual finds in this a freedom to renew one's relations with the world, and thus to recalibrate one's relations with oneself: 'The central virtue of aesthetic sensibility consists in the capacity for finding oneself through detachment from oneself' (277). With a turn of phrase reminiscent of Gawande's, Seel (who earlier in his career studied well-being) emphasizes that a free self-relationship in the aesthetic cannot be distinguished from sharing in the alterity of the artwork: 'In other words, heteronomy must be an essential dimension of autonomy, if the latter is not to decay into isolation and alienation' (275). The freedom in aesthetics, writes Seel, subsists in this dynamic of active passivity (274). As he puts it, 'aesthetic freedom is constitutive of the capacity for self-determination' (280).

My point is that the characterizations of existential health and aesthetic experience substantially overlap, and this has implications for the question of the instrumentalization of art in the field of arts and health. If one concentrates on existential health rather than any other specific health effects, then art activities in healthcare no longer appear a trivializing instrumentalization of art for external purposes, but rather a realization of the genuine essence of aesthetic experience. This argument is consolidated by findings in the field of empirical aesthetics. Empirical aesthetics differ from arts and health in its aim to examine the aesthetic experience per se, without any external objective beyond a pure search for knowledge; but unlike philosophical aesthetics, which it otherwise resembles, it relies on empirical methods with quantifiable data, as is standard in arts and health.

Empirical studies using functional magnetic resonance imaging (fMRI) at New York University and the Max Planck Institute in

Frankfurt indicate that aesthetic experiences activate the default mode network (DMN) in the brain (Vessel et al. 2013; Vessel et al. 2019). The DMN is a widespread but distinct neuronal network activated during resting wakefulness and in the spontaneous introspective states of mind that follow on it, such as mind-wandering, past and future simulations, thinking of others' mental states, and autobiographical recollections (Andrews-Hanna 2012). It is usually deactivated, though, when attention is directed to external objects and targets, at which point other neuronal systems take over. However, Vessel and colleagues found that for particularly intense aesthetic experiences—of artworks which their research subjects said affected them strongly—the deactivation of the DMN ceased, even when the subjects' attention was directed to external stimuli (the artworks). In particular, high levels of activity were noted in the medial prefrontal cortex (mPFC), the subsystem associated with mental self-representation and self-esteem. Vessel and colleagues conclude:

> We propose that certain artworks can 'resonate' with an individual's sense of self … This access [to the DMN], which other external stimuli normally do not obtain, allows the representation of the artwork to interact with the neural processes related to the self, affect them, and possibly even be incorporated into them (i.e., into the future, evolving representation of self). (Vessel et al. 2013, 6)

The results of fMRI studies thus appear to support the posited link between aesthetic experience and self-reflexivity, as theorized in philosophical aesthetics. This link, which empirical and philosophical aesthetics postulates on the basis of differing theoretical frameworks and methods—that is, different knowledge criteria—is, in turn, in line with the characterization of existential health as being conditional on autonomy and participation.

This reasoning, with its voices from different disciplines, is intended as an example of an intermediary discourse that could explore the overlaps between different fields of knowledge. Here the overlap means that the polar opposite approaches of the aesthetic disciplines and arts and health to the instrumentalization of art are brought into contact with each other and thus prompt fresh dialogue and knowledge exchange. It also demonstrates that aesthetic experiences really are epistemological boundary objects, studied in many academic fields using radically different knowledge criteria. If any intermediary discourse is to succeed, it is wise to set aside the question of the validity of each field's fundamental knowledge criteria, if only temporarily, as such discussions tend to increase their polarization (see, for example, Rampley 2017). That said, one should not expect (nor do I see it as desirable) that the tensions between views on specific issues—such as here, the instrumentalization of art—are reduced to nothing. As Seel emphasizes, good can come of an aesthetic experience—insights, changes in attitude, broader perspectives—but above all it is worthwhile in itself: 'The playgrounds of aesthetic openness are not a mere training camp in which special skills are learned' (2014, 276).

Co-production of phenomenological knowledge

Thus far I have used 'intermediary discourse' to describe a possible dialogue between the various academic fields concerned with the aesthetic experience, much as Rabeharisoa and Callon (2004 *passim*) use the term to describe communication between biomedical researchers and patients and relatives, organized in a progressive patients' association, or as Markus Idvall uses it in the present volume in studying communication between medical scientists and patients. I will now show that conversations during a visit by people with Parkinson's disease to an art museum can be regarded as intermediary discourses, leading to the co-production of knowledge in a phenomenological perspective, privileging the subjective understanding of the individual who has the experience over objectively verifiable descriptions. It should be noted that 'intermediary discourse' risks losing its analytical edge if applied in too many differing empirical circumstances. However, I would argue that the fact that it can be operationalized in different contexts is testimony to the concept's usefulness. My example is taken from a research collaboration, Presence-Oriented Art Pedagogy, with the art historian Peter Bengtsen and the ethnologist Åsa Alftberg, with the aim to develop a mediation methodology for encounters with art, which focuses on the sensation of presence rather than on interpretation of the artworks' meanings, which otherwise is a common focus of art pedagogy.[5] In the project, informed by Hans Ulrich Gumbrecht's distinction (2003) between meaning and presence as two fundamental elements in the aesthetic experience, we used a three-step method of our own making to mediate art (Appendix, Figure 8.2). In the first step, participants concentrate on the artwork, alert to their perception of it. In the second step, they describe their perceptions to the group, each making a conscious effort to listen to the others' perceptions. The third step is a deepening of their awareness of their perceptions, which comes of verbalizing their own experiences and hearing others' descriptions. A more detailed description of the method is found in the Appendix to this chapter. The method makes the most of group dynamics and the alternation between quiet contemplation and social interaction. By switching between attention to one's own perceptions and engaging in the other participants' verbal communications, the participants engaged in a playful examination of what Seel describes as 'an abundance of forms and relationships that we usually fail to recognize' (2014, 271). We saw a notable increase in the participants' involvement and initiative, both when interacting with the artworks and with one another, compared to when the same group had been to an art exhibition under more conventional conditions. The group now spent significantly longer time taking in the artworks.

The experiment addressed many aspects of perception and its verbalization, but here I limit myself to one: how statements made within the group served to co-produce knowledge, with which the participants helped one another deepen their experience of the artworks. At the Museum of Artistic Process and Public Art, Lund University's art museum, where the experiment was conducted, there is a plaster model by the British artist Henry Moore (1898–1986) for his sculpture *Hill Arches* (1973), which is now found realized in bronze in several places around the world. One photo (Appendix, Figure 8.1) shows a reconstruction of the situation with participants seated in front of Moore's model. Very little seems to be happening, but in fact they are engrossed in the first step, making themselves aware of their perception of the work.

When it was time for the second step of the method, verbalization, one participant began by saying, 'The sculpture has its dark side towards us.' It would be easy to think it a simple statement of fact, but in the context in which it was said it was above all a description of an experience. In all its simplicity, it is a blueprint for what can be called the anatomy of presence—including all its constitutive elements. There are three such elements: the artwork, the beholder, and the space that encompasses them both. The statement shows that the participant sensed their specific relationship in that situation: because of the way the light fell in the room, they were sitting in the sculpture's shadow. The participants were together on the same side of the artwork in this case—they had looked at other works from different positions—and the other participants' statements about the sculpture were to broadly the same effect: 'The sculpture is between us and the window.' 'It's blocking the light.' All of them include the work, the room, and the beholder, whether explicitly or implicitly. They thus express the fundamental phenomenological condition for the experience of presence: our body constitutes a volume in a space we share with other bodies. It brings with it a myriad of aspects and nuances for perception to explore—our project revolved around their identification and systematization for use in our mediation method.

In the present context, however, the key point was that participants built their knowledge, their awareness of perception, in dialogue with one another. In an evaluation after they had gone round the exhibition, participants stressed how valuable the group conversation had been in giving them a more profound experience. The process amounted to the participants being engaged in the co-production of phenomenological knowledge—phenomeno-logical in the sense that their statements only had meaning under the specific conditions in which they were said. Far from being a statement of objective fact—for example, 'The sculpture is white and made from plaster', which is true, regardless of who says it and where—the statements made by the participants are valid only if said right there, in the shadow of *Hill Arches*. By articulating what is in this sense phenomenological knowledge, the project's method serves to intensify the aesthetic experience.

Can art historians join in this kind of co-production of phenomenological knowledge? If so, under what circumstances? The instinctive answer is that of course they can participate, for the simple reason that art historians, like anyone else, are able (and presumably willing) to be open to aesthetic experiences. The primary condition for their participation in a phenomenological exchange of knowledge is thus that they accept their role as *participants*, and that they ascribe their subjective aesthetic experiences the status of knowledge in the framework of the intermediary discourse.[6] However, there is also a more specialized level on which the art historian's scholarship has a part to play in intermediary discourses. The aesthetic disciplines are guardians of a long legacy of knowledge about things aesthetic. The fact that this knowledge is largely separate from the field of arts and health is perhaps the most detrimental effect of the gap between the two spheres of knowledge. If the gap could be bridged it would be very useful, especially for the reflexive element in arts and health activities. For example, the art historian Alois Riegl (1858–1905), one of the significant figures of the discipline, used his book on group portraits in Dutch art in the seventeenth century (1999 [1902/1931]) to develop the formalist approach for which he is known into a theory that relies on the beholder's relation to the artwork and the artwork's appeal to the beholder. He saw the beholder and artwork as joined in a mutual recognition, because the beholder has a sense, as an element embedded in his aesthetic consideration, that the artwork is looking back at him. As Margaret Olin (1989, 295) notes, Riegl's views were not far removed from his contemporary Edmund Husserl (1859–1938) and his phenom-enological philosophy, or indeed Martin Buber (1878–1965) and his theological theories of intersubjectivity in what he termed the I–Thou relationship. This mutual attentiveness (*Aufmerksamkeit*, a term Riegl operationalizes) is notably free from what Margaret Iversen calls 'egotistic isolation' (1993, 94), and rather is suffused by fundamental respect for the other (Riegl 1999, 313) as well as self-respect—here Olin (1989, 291) reminds us that the term respect comes from the Latin *respicere*, to look back.

This notion—that in aesthetic receptivity there is an element of being addressed or 'seen' by the artwork—articulates something we noticed in conversation as the participants went round the exhibition, albeit only as hints rather than fully formulated reflections. That is where art history could help with the co-production of phenomenological knowledge, linking what the participants are hinting at to the corresponding elements in the history of aesthetic thought. It could offer the cognitive and conceptual tools with which to express experience in words. This sort of articulation could strengthen people's reflexive awareness of this component of the aesthetic experience, which as far as the project is concerned amounts to the method's third step, to deepen the experience.

Shared or different goals
when co-producing knowledge

Another example from the history of aesthetic thought that could enrich the field of arts and health is what is sometimes referred to as the West's first aesthetic theory, which is also a theory of love. In Plato's *Symposium* (*c.*385–370 BC), he has Socrates summarize the teachings of the priestess Diotima of Mantinea in what is known as the Ladder of Love (Plato 2001, 210a–212d). Diotima had explained that one who loves will learn the nature of beauty step by step, first by discovering the beauty of a single body, then in another body that is different from the first, and so on in an ever-increasing circle from the specific to the abstract, until finally seeing beauty itself:

> beginning from these beautiful things here, always to proceed on
> up for the sake of that beauty, using these beautiful things here as
> steps: from one to two, and from two to all beautiful bodies; and
> from beautiful bodies to beautiful pursuits; and from pursuits to
> beautiful lessons; and from lessons to end at that lesson, which
> is the lesson of nothing else than the beautiful itself; and at last
> to know what is beauty itself. (211b–c)

How can an account written two and a half thousand years ago, and which ranges from physical homosexual desire to the divine, shed light on modern experiences of art in healthcare contexts? To answer that question we must first look at the related issue of what art history has to forego in order to join in an intermediary discourse of this kind. For Rabeharisoa and Callon, an intermediary discourse is an organized communication in which no party's perspective is allowed to dominate (in their example, neither the researchers' 'technical' nor the patient organization's 'strategic' perspectives). Each party thus has to sacrifice something from their own sphere of knowledge. The aesthetic disciplines are in the habit of thinking about aesthetic theories, such as Riegl's or Plato's, framed by the broad metaphysical frameworks or world views of the historical contexts where the theories took shape. Riegl devised his reception theory, *avant la lettre*, from his historicist view of artistic idiom as an expression of national temperament; Diotima's Ladder of Love was based in Plato's Theory of Forms. Understanding the thinking about aesthetics in the light of its historical context is central to the history of art. But this is precisely what I would argue art history has to abstain from to a certain extent, if only provisionally and tactically, if it is to have a part in the intermediary discourse sketched here. Instead, art history should hold up a phenomenological lens to aesthetic theories, seeing them as descriptions of experiences. Seen thus, Diotima's Ladder was not just Plato's way of expressing his Theory of Forms; it was a conceptualization of a certain aspect of aesthetic experience, an aspect which manifested in the art activity for people with Parkinson's referred to above. It is found in the tendency for the focus of aesthetic attentiveness to be transferred from a single object to several, and extending to take in the full scope of artwork–beholder–space, accompanied by an intensification or consolidation of the aesthetic experience. Like Riegl's theory, Diotima's Ladder of Love can be a cognitive tool with which to articulate a particular facet of experience that might be difficult to put into words otherwise—in this case, in the image of upward movement, towards a high vantage point with a wider horizon, from where one can see more. Such articulations can strengthen the reflexive element and help the mediation method develop.

If art history makes a concession—putting the historical metaphysical frameworks to one side—to participate in an intermediary discourse, it can only be on a temporary, provisional basis in order to achieve a strategic goal in the field of arts and health. Historical contextualization is fundamental to the aesthetic disciplines' sphere of knowledge, and cannot be abandoned. That is why I hold that Bommenel's hypothesis, that any interdisciplinary research requires all its researchers to agree on a shared vision of their research goals, has to be nuanced. Research can have several goals, and not all of them need to apply in all circumstances. An example of a shared goal could be co-producing knowledge about the potential of the aesthetic experience in healthcare, but alongside that, the field of arts and health and the aesthetic disciplines could have different goals and research questions, rooted in their respective spheres of knowledge. For arts and health, it might be 'How can we use the arts to improve the lives of the elderly and the sick?' For the aesthetic disciplines, meanwhile, 'What do such art activities teach us about the aesthetic experience?'

Notes

1   For overviews see, for example, Sigurdson 2014; Sjölander & Sigurdson 2016; Crossick & Kaszynska 2016; and APPGAHW 2017.
2   See also WHO 2019.
3   Other things than art, such as nature or sport, can also offer an aesthetic experience of course, and far from all art has an aesthetic experience as its goal. My purpose

here is not to cover all the meanings of the concept, but rather to address a specific problem on which the concept has some bearing.

4 *Constitution of the World Health Organization*, p. 1. The Constitution was adopted at the International Health Conference in New York, 17 June to 22 July 1946, and came into force on 7 April 1948.

5 The project's original name was 'Systematic implementation of aesthetic experiences and artistic activities in the care of persons with Parkinson's disease', and was part of BAGADILICO, the Basal Ganglia Disorders Linnaeus Consortium, funded by the Swedish Research Council (2008–2018). See also Alftberg & Rosenqvist 2017; Rosenqvist & Suneson 2016; Mittelman & Epstein 2009; and Rosenberg et al. 2009.

6 This might prompt in some practitioners a worry of the kind that has stalked the discipline since its inception concerning its legitimacy as *Wissenschaft* and the risk of being considered too subjective (see Rampley 2011).

References

Alftberg, Åsa & Johanna Rosenqvist (2017), 'Meetings with complexity: Dementia and participation in art educational situations', in Kristofer Hansson & Markus Idvall (eds.), *Interpreting the brain in society: Cultural reflections on neuroscientific practices* (Lund: Arkiv Förlag).

Andrews-Hanna, Jessica R. (2012), 'The brain's default network and its adaptive role in internal mentation', *The Neuroscientist*, 18,(3), 251–70.

APPGAHW (2017), *Creative health: The arts for health and wellbeing* (Inquiry report, All-Party Parliamentary Group on Arts, Health and Wellbeing).

Bommenel, Elin (2012), 'Credibility and legitimacy: Challenges to interdisciplinary research', in Max Liljefors, Susanne Lundin & Andréa Wiszmeg (eds.), *The atomized body: The cultural life of stem cells, genes and neurons* (Lund: Nordic Academic Press).

Crossick, Geoffrey & Patrycja Kaszynska (2016), *Understanding the value of arts & culture* (AHRC Cultural Value Project; Swindon: Arts & Humanities Research Council).

Danto, Arthur (1997), *After the end of art: Contemporary art and the pale of history* (Princeton: PUP).

Fancourt, Daisy & Saoirse Finn (2019), *What is the evidence on the role of the arts in improving health and well-being? A scoping review* (Health Evidence Network synthesis report 67; WHO).

Gawande, Atul (2014), *Being mortal: Illness, medicine and what matters in the end* (London: Profile).

Greenberg, Clement (1982 [1965]), 'Modernist painting', in Francis Franscina & Charles Harrison (eds.), *Modern art and modernism: A critical anthology* (New York: Harper & Row).

Gumbrecht, Hans Ulrich (2003), *Production of presence: What meaning cannot convey* (Palo Alto: Stanford University Press).

Hyun, Insoo (2016), 'The surprising complexities of stem cell medical travel', in Susanne Lundin, Charlotte Kroløkke, Michael N. Petersen & Elmi Muller (eds.), *Global bodies in grey zones: Health, hope, biotechnology* (Stellenbosch: SUN MeDIA & STIAS).

Iversen, Margaret (1993), *Alois Riegl: Art history and theory* (Cambridge, MA: MIT Press).

Jasanoff, Sheila (2004a), 'The idiom of co-production', in ead. (ed.), *States of knowledge: The co-production of science and social order* (London: Routledge).

—— (2004b), 'Ordering knowledge, ordering society", in ead. (ed.), *States of knowledge: The co-production of science and social order* (London: Routledge).

Kant, Immanuel (2002), *Critique of the power of judgment* (Cambridge: CUP) (first pub. as *Kritik der Urteilskraft*, 1790).

Liljefors, Max & Åsa Alftberg (2019), *Konst som resurs i geriatrisk vård: Rapport från ett följeforskningsprojekt om Resa i tid och rum—En konstvandring på Nacka sjukhus* (Stockholm: Region Stockholm).

Melder, Cecilia (2011), *Vilsenhetens Epidemiologi: En religionspsykologisk studie i existentiell hälsa* (Acta Universitatis Upsaliensis, Psychologia et sociologia religionum 25; Uppsala: UUP).

Mittelman, Mary & Epstein, Cynthia (2009), 'Evaluation of meet me at MoMA', in Rosenberg, Francesca, Amir Parsa, Laurel Humble & Carrie McGee (2009) (eds.), *meetme: Making art accessible to people with dementia* (New York: Museum of Modern Art).

Olin, Margaret (1989), 'Forms of respect: Alois Riegl's concept of attentiveness', *Art Bulletin*, 71(2), 285–99.

Plato (2001), *Plato's Symposium: A Translation by Seth Benardete with commentaries by Allan Bloom and Seth Benardete* (Chicago: University of Chicago Press).

Priebe, Gunilla & Morten Sager (2014), 'Konst och hälsa', in Ola Sigurdson (ed.), *Kultur och hälsa: Ett vidgat perspektiv* (Gothenburg: Göteborgs universitet, Centrum för kultur och hälsa).

Rabeharisoa, Vololona & Michel Callon (2004), 'Patients and scientists in French muscular dystrophy research', in Sheila Jasanoff (ed.), *States of knowledge: The co-production of science and social order* (London: Routledge).

Rampley, Matthew (2011), 'The idea of a scientific discipline: Rudolf von Eitelberger and the emergence of art history in Vienna, 1847–1873', *Art History*, 34 (1), 54–79.

—— (2017), *The seductions of Darwin: Art, evolution, neuroscience* (Pennsylvania: Pennsylvania State University Press).

Riegl, Alois (1999), *The group portraiture of Holland*, introduction by W. Kemp, tr. E. M. Kain & D. Britt (Los Angeles: Getty Research Institute for the History of Art and the Humanities) (first pub. *Das holländische Gruppenporträt*, 1902/1931).

Rosenberg, Francesca, Amir Parsa, Laurel Humble & Carrie McGee (2009) (eds.), *Meetme: Making art accessible to people with dementia* (New York: Museum of Modern Art).

Rosenqvist, Johanna & Ellen Suneson (2016), 'Konst och subjektskapande: Neurodegenerativa nedsättningar och dialogbaserad konstpedagogik', *Socialmedicinsk tidskrift*, 3, 288–96.

Seel, Martin (2014), 'Active passivity: On the aesthetic variant of treedom', *Estetika: The Central European Journal of Aesthetics*, 51(2), 269–81.

Sigurdson, Ola (2014), 'Introduktion till kultur och hälsa', in Ola Sigurdson (ed.), *Kultur och hälsa: Ett vidgat perspektiv* (Gothenburg: Centrum för kultur och hälsa, Göteborgs universitet).

Sjölander, Annica & Ola Sigurdson (2016), preface in eid. (eds.), *Kultur och hälsa i praktiken* (Gothenburg: Centrum för kultur och hälsa, Göteborgs universitet).

Star, Susan & James Griesemer (1989), 'Ecology, "translations" and boundary objects: Amateurs and professionals in Berkeley's Museum of vertebrate zoology, 1907–39', *Social Studies of Science*, 19(3), 387–420.

Temel, Jennifer S., et al. (2010), 'Early palliative care for patients with metastatic non-small-cell lung cancer', *New England Journal of Medicine*, 363(8), 733–42.

Vessel, Edward A., et al. (2019), 'The default-mode network represents aesthetic appeal that generalizes across visual domains', *Proceedings of the National Academy of Sciences*, 116(38), 19155–64.

——, Gabrielle G. Starr & Nava Rubin (2013), 'Art reaches within: Aesthetic experience, the self and the default mode network', *Frontiers in Neuroscience*, 7 (art. 258), 1–9.

WHO (2006 [1946]), *Constitution of the World Health Organization: Basic documents* (45th edn, New York: WHO).

WHO Regional Office of Europe (2019), *Intersectoral action: The arts, health and well-being* (Sector brief on Arts).

Appendix

Presence-oriented art pedagogy

The purpose of the project Presence-oriented art pedagogy is to develop a method for the mediation of art, which privileges experiences of presence over interpretation of the artwork's symbolic meanings.

Summary

The project develops a novel method of art pedagogy that combines results from our own experiments in mediation with insights from aesthetic philosophy. The project applies a phenomenological perspective to aesthetic philosophy, which means that the focus is not metaphysical frameworks, but expressions of experience. The starting point is the distinction made by the literary scholar Hans Ulrich Gumbrecht between meaning and presence as two basic elements in encounters with art. To interpret an artwork's meaning is basically to explain it intellectually, in reference to, for example, the artist's intentions, the work's historical context, or the beholder's associations. Most art pedagogy revolves around this kind of interpretation. To explore an artwork's presence is instead to become aware of one's perceptual sensations of the work here-and-now. The project's method does not preclude interpretation, but is nevertheless primarily concerned with the experience of presence. The project members have observed greater initiative and commitment from participants in the experiments with a presence-oriented method.

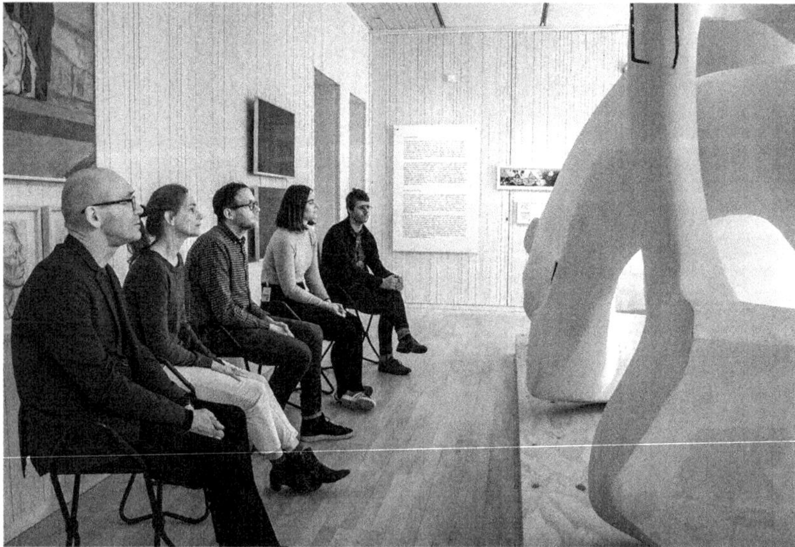

Figure 8.1. Participants are looking at Henry Moore's Hill Arches (1973) at the Musuem of Artistic Process and Public Art in Lund. They are paying attention to their perceptions of the sculpture, in Step 1 of the pedagogical model. (The photo shows a reconstruction.) Photographer: Peter Bengtsen.

I

Method

The method is a three-step model (Figure 8.2).

In the first step, participants alert themselves to their own perceptions of an artwork. In the second step, they verbalize their sensations by describing them to the other participants, and listen to the others' verbalizations. The third step is the intensified experience that results from the verbalizations, which in turn can be the subject of keen awareness, and so the cycle begins again. The method uses the rhythm struck up between the individual participant's silent attentiveness to the artwork and the social exchange between participants.

Artwork–beholder–space

'The sculpture has its dark side towards us.'

This statement by one of the participants, sitting looking at Henry Moore's Hill Arches (Figure 8.1), articulates their sensation of the artwork in the here and now, representing a phenomenological knowledge that is only valid in the place and at the time it is uttered—in the shadow of the sculpture as sunlight shone through the window. It also contains all three key components of the experience of presence: the artwork, the beholder, and the space they share.

What does phenomenological knowledge 'feel' like compared to objective knowledge? The reader can find out by looking at the image of Hill Arches (Figure 8.3) while thinking 'The sculpture is white and made from plaster'—an objective statement which is correct

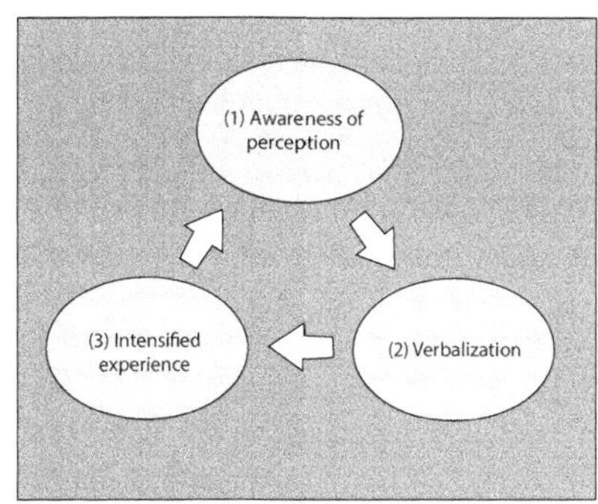

Figure 8.2. Three-step pedagogical method for the mediation of art.

regardless of where and when it is said. Then look at it again and think 'The sculpture's sunlit side is towards me.' For some, this statement (which expresses phenomenological know-ledge) gives them a sense that the artwork addresses them, even though their perception of it is mediated through a photograph.

Aesthetic experience

People have created art for tens of thousands of years. And for thousands of years they have formulated philosophical theories about the aesthetic experience. One eternal theme is that an aesthetic experience can be deeply satisfying and empowering. It can also be associated with feelings of love and gratitude. In recent years, academic studies have shown that aesthetic experiences can have many types of measurable, positive effects on health and well-being. The WHO recommends that art's healing, strengthening, and rehabilitative potential should be systematically integrated into the WHO's European Health Policy.

Active passivity, or, the free play of perception and cognition

An important thought in the philosophy of aesthetics is that in any aesthetic experience the individual's perception and cognition can play freely. Aesthetic attentiveness is not limited by expectations of how things should be perceived or what that should lead to. Therefore, the aesthetic experience is characterized by a greater sense of the here-and-now, leaving it open for the individual to notice forms and relationships overlooked in a normal frame of mind. It creates an inner freedom unique to the aesthetic experience. This, in turn, can give the viewer a renewed sense of self, as someone who can have these perceptions, who appreciates these nuances, who sees these relationships in which he himself has a part. In this way, an aesthetic experience can reinforce the viewer's inner autonomy. The philosopher Martin Seel calls the aesthetic approach 'active passivity', for as attention goes it is deliberately elicited, matched by a readiness to fully accept what the work of art can give.

Universal parameters

Within the triad of artwork–beholder–space are a number of variables that factor into perception. They have been taken as the universal parameters for the project, because they are a feature of almost every aesthetic situation. Examples include colour, form, the play of light and shadow, and variations in distance, size, and spatial direction. Perception as such also has its variables, such as broad or narrow attentiveness, or a focus on specific characteristics and qualities. All such parameters can be used to vary and increase the individual's awareness of perception, and are therefore useful tools in any presence-oriented pedagogy.

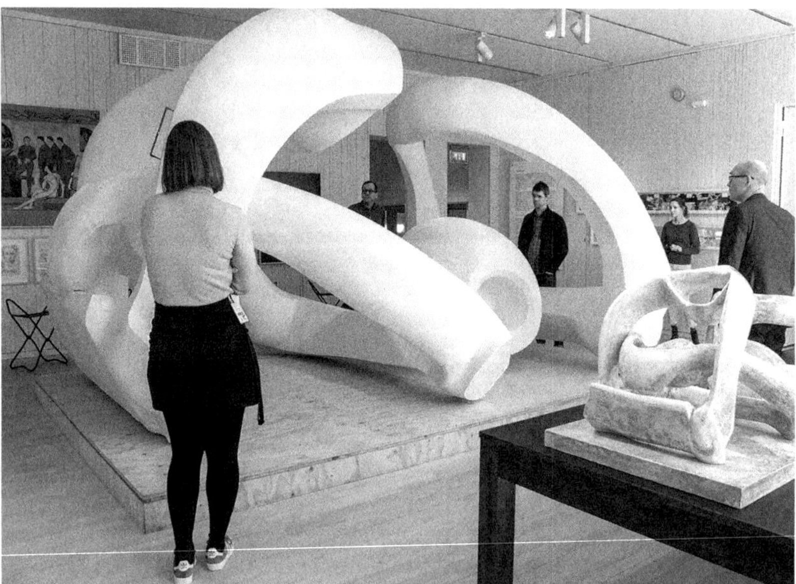

Figure 8.3. When the particpants take in the artwork from different positions, their perceptions of the artwork–beholder–space relation will differ. As they verbalize their experiences for one another, a dynamic shift in perceptions can take place. (The photo shows a reconstruction.) Photographer: Peter Bengtsen.

The play of light and shadow

Looking at Carl Eldh's models for a sculpture of August Strindberg (Figure 8.4), one participant burst out 'How beautifully the light falls on the sculptures!' When the researchers asked the group to describe what they could see, the participants found it difficult to put it into words at first, perhaps because the scene is complex, with several free-standing figures. When asked to focus on what was lightest, however, they began by pointing out the parts of the sculptures which were in full sunlight. Then they went on to identify the darkest parts, which lay in the deepest shadow. From there, they went on to explore the nuances in between, the parts that are not so easily defined as 'light' or 'dark'. The group were engaged in this exercise for over 30 enthusiastic minutes. It is an example of how the method uses specific parameters—in this case, light and shadow—to open up and consolidate the individual's awareness of sensation.

Imaginative power

In aesthetic philosophy, there is always a sense in which the human imagination—or, as it is also called, imaginative power (Kant's Einbildungskraft)—has a key role in many mental processes. It revolves around the ability to create and maintain an image or idea as an inner vision, ostensibly assembling the beholder's impressions into a coherent representation in the beholder's mind. Looking at an Andy Goldsworthy installation (Figure 8.5), the participants' perceptions alternated between a number of such coherent 'imaginings'. For example, the installation's bulrushes were seen as forming a porous membrane, which divided the space into two different 'light rooms'; or as a wall with an opening in the middle; or as dashes, the traces of movement through the air, criss-crossing in all directions; or frozen in the moment of tumbling down. These imaginings centre on different parameters, whether light–shadow or direction, and so on. The transitions between them are spontaneous, since the

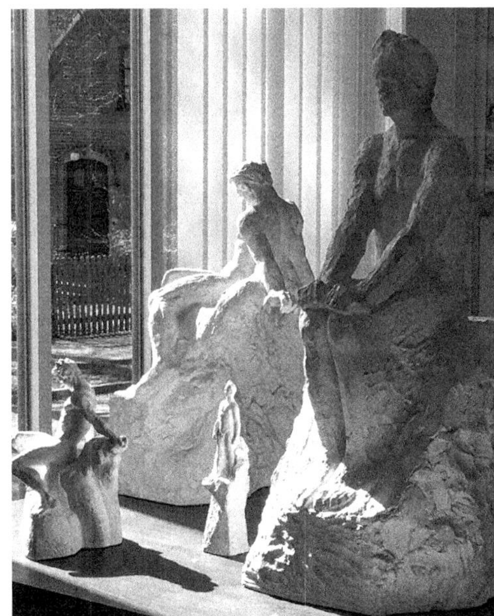

Figure 8.4. Models for Carl Eldh's monument of August Strindberg, erected in Tegnérlunden park in Stockholm in 1942. The Museum of Artistic Process and Public Art, Lund. Photographer: Max Liljefors.

imaginative power of the aesthetic is free, and not dictated by logic or utility. None of these images are right or wrong, true or false. The imagination can also include the beholder, because the individual's aesthetic attentiveness turns outwards, towards the work of art, and inwards, towards one's own perceptions and cognition. The beholder feels that new perceptual and cognitive ideas take shape in the encounter with the artwork. Carl Eldh's figures gave one participant the impression that the smallest sculpture was in fact huge. She saw herself standing in front of it, looking up at it (though in reality she was standing where the photo had been taken), and this gave her the feeling of looking at the scene from a long way off. This made participants aware of the difference between physical and perceived distance, another parameter in the project's method. Participants could even imagine their own gaze as an invisible hand, with which they could reach out and touch the artworks.

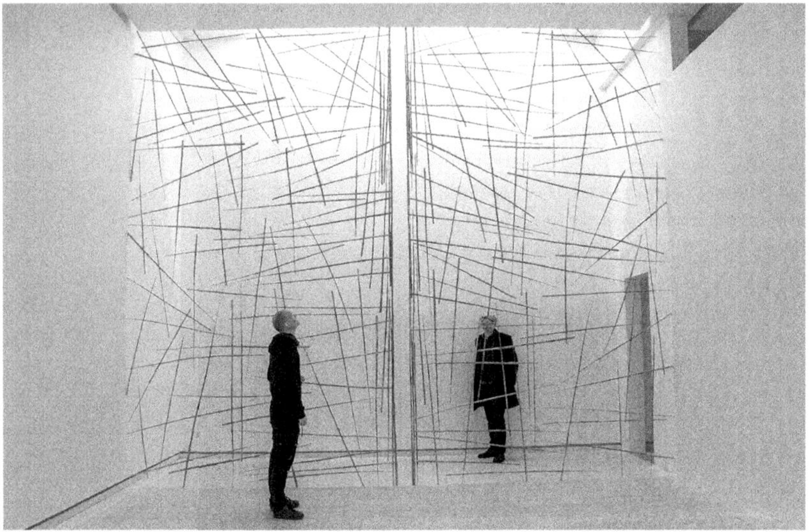

Figure 8.5. Installation by Andy Goldsworthy, 2017–2018, at the Museum of Artistic Process and Public Art, Lund. Photographer: Peter Bengtsen.

The project Presence-Oriented Art Pedagogy started as part of the Linnaeus research programme BAGADILICO, Basal Ganglia Disorders Linnaeus Consortium, at Lund University, funded by the Swedish Research Council 2008–2018. BAGADILICO was a multi-disciplinary research programme uniting researchers from the medical, technological and humanistic faculties at Lund University, in research about Huntington's and Parkinson's diseases. Today, Presence-Oriented Art Pedagogy continues as a collaboration between the Research node for Medical Humanities and the Research node for Aesthetic Studies at the Department of Arts and Cultural Sciences, Lund University.

V

CHAPTER 9

Medicines in the grey market

A sociocultural analysis of individual agency

Rui Liu & Susanne Lundin

> Therefore, I prefer to get medicines myself so I have the opportunity to check the quality… In this way, I can ensure that no dangerous chemical stuff is used in the production process. My doctor knows I'm using cannabis, instead of the one he can prescribe which only worsens my condition.

This quote comes from our study *Where and how do you buy medicines?*[1] The respondent has been consuming cannabis for twelve years, claiming it works well to manage his pain. One way to obtain cannabis is to get family to send it from abroad. Cannabis consumption is not a common healing practice among our respondents. However, between the lines, this respondent articulates a complex yet increasingly common view of medicines and how to access them in contemporary society. Somehow, it hints at a desire to gain some control over one's body, by skilfully distinguishing what are considered as good medicines from bad ones. Such practice is often characterized as self-care, as opposed to care provided by medical professionals. Furthermore, suggested in this quote is the emergence of an array of relations: markets entering institutions, self-care constituting public care, and lay perspectives encountering professional ones. Alongside, individual agency is taking shape.

Health systems, in Sweden as elsewhere, are often conceptualized as 'knowledge economies that produce and mediate access to health knowledge embedded in people, services and commodities' (Bloom et al. 2008, 2077). Although medicines are commonly perceived as desirable and valuable things to transform the body, they may cause harm if handled improperly. The consumption of medicines is thus usually subject to many legal restrictions. Between people and medicines, there often stand medical professionals, whose institutional expertise allow them to act as medicine gatekeepers. Therefore, in the interaction of people and medicines at various stages from production to consumption, during and beyond clinical encounters, knowledge is materialized and mobilized in the form of the medicines. It means that knowledge can also be understood as a praxis or a form of doing. Following this line of thought, in the case of medicines knowledge does not merely represent awareness about how to take care of one's body, but it denotes a set of skills obtained through everyday consumption praxis. In this chapter, we use this to investigate how knowledge as a praxis is intertwined with consumption in everyday life. We situate our discussion in the Swedish setting, while remaining attuned to the global phenomenon that is the spread of poor-quality medicines on the market.

Setting the scene

In 2009, Sweden witnessed a shift in its retail pharmaceutical landscape. A liberal pharmacy market replaced forty years of state-owned monopoly, Apoteket AB, and its nationwide control of drug supplies. Private suppliers were allowed to enter the market, and some over-the-counter (OTC) medicines can now be bought elsewhere than pharmacies. To further increase service efficiency, many kinds of digitalized healthcare services are now available to the public. Take an example, as of autumn 2015 all authorized Swedish pharmacies can sell medicines and medical advice online. Although online medicine purchases are much easier than ever before, this loosely regulated virtual market dissolves national borders and opens up for unauthorized provision of medicines. Unlicensed online pharmacies spring up, and a majority of them, if not all, offer consumers unrestricted access to all kinds of medical products, including prescription-only medicines (POM), whose therapeutic quality cannot be guaranteed (Clark 2015; Liang & Mackey 2012). Even more worrying for the Swedish authorities, at the other end of the supply chain there are signs showing that increasing numbers of Swedish residents are buying medicines from unauthorized channels (Swedish Medical Products Agency 2015). On the global scale, the trade in illicit medicines in the grey market is expanding tremendously, harming individuals and society (Newton et al. 2016). This affects all countries in the world and infiltrates all marketplaces, whether online or offline, formal or informal (Nayyar et al. 2019). To tackle this public health threat, national and international stakeholders have called for collaboration. To facilitate collaborations, in May 2017 the WHO launched a working definition of these dangerous medicines—substandard and falsified (SF) medical products (WHO 2017).

In the current literature on the phenomenon of SF medical products, studies in medicine, law, and public health have led the way. Much of the focus is on the supply side, advocating technological innovation and harmonized international legal frameworks (Attaran 2015; Liu & Lundin 2016; Rebiere et al. 2017). Consumer perspectives, however, are usually omitted. When individuals are mentioned, they are often portrayed as either vulnerable victims or naïve consumers who risk their lives to buy medicines outside the legal market. Certainly, practical issues such as accessibility and affordability are important determining factors in the decision-making process, especially among populations with financial constraints (Alfadl et al. 2013; Nordstrom 2007). For this reason, welfare states like Sweden, with an established and functioning public healthcare system and nationwide healthcare insurance coverage, the increasingly common practice of buying medicines illicitly is intriguing.

A number of criminological studies in the British context provide some insights which account for this illicit act. They point to the direct link between the demand for medicines in general, the widespread availability of illicit medical products, and often invisible grey markets (for example, Hall & Antonopoulos 2016; Sugiura 2018). Nonetheless, the transition from demand to practice, meaning here the consumption of medicines, is not always straightforward. For example, buyers' trust in informal drug sellers could be interpreted as a guarantee of medicine quality, as shown in a study of migrant buyers in South Africa (Hornberger & Cossa 2012). Or, as found in a UK study (Sugiura et al. 2012), a sense of entitlement may become the consumers' argument for moving to the extra-legal market, regardless of the medicines' legal status. Implied in these studies is that demand is expressed through different forms of consumption strategy. And essentially, all such strategies are relational and contextual. Linking back to the portrayal of consumers in the literature on SF medical products, we argue that dichotomizing between passive victims and autonomous agents neither helps to explain *why* people buy medicines illicitly, nor does it elucidate *how* grey markets take form (see Gunnarson & Lundin 2015). On this account, by tracing the connections between knowledge as a form of doing and everyday consumption, we offer an alternative analysis of individual agency and various expressions of demand.

Researching medicines

Our primary source material is a survey comprising 155 answers from Swedish residents, collected by the authors in April and May 2016 with the assistance of Lund University's Folklife Archives. We also draw on results from netnographic observations conducted by another project member shortly after the survey (Brissman 2016). The data were coded as themes emerged and then categorized accordingly. Respondents have been anonymized to avoid identification. We would argue that the respondents' answers serve as a keyhole to a larger research stream about grey markets. Notably, the patterns we identify in this chapter are not unique in the phenomenon of SF medical products. The search for alternatives in the grey zones and the victim–agent dichotomy are not unusual themes in studies of other socio-medical phenomena such as medical travel. In our analysis, we thus draw on insights from those studies to strengthen our arguments.

We begin by introducing two analytical concepts—liquid consumption and prosumption—with which we explore how consumption strategies reveal the enactment of agency and the movement of knowledge. The presentation of our findings and analysis is organized around three medicine-purchasing scenarios, each centred on a specific type of object: prescriptions in medical consultations, the logo of legal online pharmacies, and medical solutions that seem promising but are only available outside the legal market.

Liquidity and prosumption

Essentially, medicines are things attributed with social and symbolic meaning (Whyte et al. 2002). Their thinginess not only gives medicines a tangible shape and texture, but concretizes various types of dysphoria so that both healthcare receivers and providers can focus their efforts. This thinginess thus also allows medicines to stand on their own, independent from medical professionals and their expertise. This means they are not only the subject of medical consultations; they can also stay with patients afterwards in the form of prescriptions (Whyte et al. 2002). This independency leads to another layer of the thinginess, which lies in that medicines can move, locally and globally, beyond clinical settings to be exchanged as commodities. In that movement, they may enter and exit various forms of markets, transcend national borders, and bridge dialogues with people and between people.

Starting off as manmade objects with the potential to cure, medicines are treated with a variety of contrasting, yet coexisting, attitudes and health beliefs such as hope and fear, trust and distrust, safe and dangerous, demand and resistance—even as generally good and bad. In turn, they also influence and shape people's experiences and expectations in terms of how and where they should be accessed and consumed (Lock & Nguyen 2010). During this interactive process, agency—the power to act—is enacted. Ideological notions of how people understand knowledge and authority need to be revisited. Liquidity, or rather the potential to become freer agents in loosely bonded relationships, emerges as a very relevant aspect.

The first concept is *liquid consumption*, proposed by Fleura Bardhi and Giana Eckhardt (2017). Rooted in Zygmunt Bauman's theory of liquid modernity (2000), liquid consumption is characterized as access-based, ephemeral, and dematerialized, in contrast to solid consumption, which is ownership-based, enduring and materialized. These two kinds of consumption coexist on a spectrum in the consumption experience. They intertwine yet remain distinguishable. In liquid consumption, the accessibility to products or services is attributed greater value than their possession. This fluidity 'enables individuals to be flexible and highly adaptable to the unpredictable demands of global mobility, economy, and labour markets' (Bardhi & Eckhardt 2017, 589). Quick circulation and immediate access are therefore emphasized in this form of consumption process. The use value and practical benefits of a product or service are prioritized over any social value. This redefined value-creation process implies that individuals may relate to social structures temporarily or only in a specific context. Another distinctive quality of liquid consumption practice is that individuals are inclined to form networks and mobilize resources within them. It differs from solid consumption, where one is more dependent on a particular channel to access services, products, or information.

The second concept is *prosumption*. Originally coined by Alvin Toffler in his book *The Third Wave* (1980), prosumption blurs production and consumption, and is historically framed by technological advances and the adoption of a neoliberal political-economic philosophy (Comor 2011). However, prosumption, like its derivative prosumer, remained unproblematized until very recently. Duly packaged, it has been embraced by marketers as a new form of civilization that frees individuals from immobility, heavy dependence on human relations, and suppression by explicit power relations. Prosumers are assumed to be imbued with creativity and autonomy by dint of their participation in such activities as self-surveillance, self-help, and sharing. Nonetheless, as Edward Comor (2011, 322) argues, without fundamental changes in the political, cultural and economic structures, individuals who actively participate in any form of prosumption will almost always 'serve status quo interests' and remain exploited by what George Ritzer (2015) terms 'prosumer capitalism'.

The concepts of liquid consumption and prosumption have useful implications for understanding why people buy medicines illegitimately. They provide us with the language and analytical angles to chart emerging consumption practices and the formation of grey markets in relation to the spread of illicit medicines. We apply these concepts here to examine how assumedly solid social norms which order everyday consumption are fluid in actual social conditions.

Multiple authorities and networked knowledge

A medical prescription is an important object that amplifies the division of roles between medical professionals and lay individuals (Whyte et al. 2002). On the practical level, it often is the tangible outcome of a medical consultation, and a legitimate proof to access certain restricted medicines. When asked about whom to consult when a prescription is needed, 'doctors' is the answer from the majority of our respondents.[2] But then this is followed by some confusion. To the rhetorical question 'How would you get a prescription-only medicine otherwise?', our respondents acknowledge not only doctors' authoritative status, but also the unavoidable part doctors play if one wants to obtain POMs legally. What is also implied is a recognition of the asymmetries between patients and doctors, in the sense that respondents position themselves as being dependent on doctors' expertise and institutional legitimacy for access to medicines. One respondent further explains:

> The very meaning of the word 'prescription' is associated with some regulations of access to medicines, right?… No matter

what, it is important, I think, to contact doctors, especially if it is about, for example, antibiotics whose use should be restrictive. In other situations, it is still important to discuss things like side effects and interaction with other medicines.

This respondent understands that one should be careful with antibiotics and taking several medicines at the same time. By articulating this, she demonstrates a certain level of medical knowledge, precisely by admitting a lack of expertise in drug use. Quite a number of respondents also mention that doctors can check up on patients' allergies and medical history to ensure the safe consumption of certain medicines. Accordingly, it is the patients' expectation that doctors act as gatekeepers, applying their expertise to minimize the potential risks and to select the right medicines for patients.

However, being dependent is not equivalent to taking a less powerful position. Whenever a respondent talks of having discussed a medical condition with their doctor, an equal and interactive relationship is depicted. A medical consultation is then turned into a conversation about the body and its subjective emotions. Thus, the doctor–patient dialogue is transformed into one between two forms of knowledge—the lay and the professional—and between two forms of care—self-care and public care (see Idvall in this volume). Instead of one party to the conversation automatically being in possession of absolute knowledge and power over the other, each contributes what they know about the body in order to formulate a treatment (although the body may have different meanings in this context, from a medical body for the doctor to an experienced body for the patient, see Mol 2002). On this account, a prescription is not simply an instruction, issued by doctors to tell patients what medications to take; it is also an individualized plan to treat the illness, and a type of contract endorsed by both patient and doctor. Thus, prescriptions can be thought of as the outcome of an embodied and emotional negotiation; a negotiation underpinned by the individual's self-reflexivity, in Anthony Giddens's term (1991, 218), accepting and presenting one's own body as 'a site of interaction, appropriation and reappropriation' where different forms of knowledge convene.

Some respondents take a relatively active part in medical consultations. For example, one respondent says that she usually prepares before visiting a doctor: 'I often first read on my own and then leave a request for a medicine.' Another respondent reflects on what happens after the visit, explaining that 'I want to know what the doctor recommends, but then I'm not sure I'll do exactly as he or she advises. But I consider it before I make my decision.' Seeing a doctor is thus thought a legitimate approach, but there is a tendency to view doctors as counsellors, whose medical advice functions as an additional input or a second opinion. In this context, prescriptions do not hold much authority as contracts any more, because they leave so much room for patients to appropriate the knowledge for their own ends. In shaping a final consumption decision, information from various sources is brought into the process to evaluate doctors' expertise. For instance, one respondent says 'I like it when the pharmacist says the same thing as the doctor. Then one knows the information is reliable'. The opinions of family and friends also play a role, as many respondents note, as do the so-called medical experts on the Internet (Brissman 2016). Gustav Brissman's netnographic observation (2016) finds that in online chatrooms some anonymous people are often regarded as medical experts, whose opinions are much valued by other members of the forum.

In the case of our survey respondents, we do not know whether they consulted people in these virtual chatrooms, but what is clearly mapped out nonetheless is a network where multiple authorities coexist. In this network, there is a range of online and offline, formal and informal actors, mediated by medicines. In our material, these actors include doctors, nurses, pharmacists, anonymous online medical experts, even non-fiction books and social media. Rather than selecting one trusted authority, what our respondents are trying to do is to evaluate and integrate different types of knowledge gained through consumption praxis before they make a decision.

Going one step further, what emerges is a dispersed yet relational network where knowledge is mobilized and prosumed. Bauman (2000) points out that the expression of numerous authorities itself presents a contradiction, in that these authorities tend to compete and counteract one another's power and influence. In the end, it is 'by the courtesy of the chooser that a would-be authority becomes an authority' (64). In the context of healthcare, laypeople are often framed as oppressed or passive, largely due to an imbalance in the possession of medical insight. Knowledge possessed by the (medical) authorities is usually deemed naturally superior. However, the respondents in our study do not merely take in knowledge from multiple sources in a network, they also synthesize it with their own understanding of the body. In this process, the information asymmetries in doctor–patient encounters are what motivates laypeople to approach the professionals for their expertise. Through the enactment of individual agency, knowledge becomes the object of prosumption.

In contrast to the majority who believe it is necessary to consult medical professionals for POMs, some respondents, however, feel disappointed with the current healthcare system. One respondent still goes to doctors' appointments for medical consultations and prescriptions, but her trust in medical expertise is low. She describes one instance when a doctor let her down.

> The doctor offered to give me penicillin 'if I wanted', even though that doctor had found a viral infection in my body. Strange but true. It lowered my trust in the profession's capabilities, not least about antibiotic resistance.

Such an experience forces her to re-evaluate the healthcare service and how to relate to doctors, not only because that particular doctor wanted to treat a viral infection with antibiotics, but because the doctor was ready to prescribe whatever medicines the respondent asked for. The doctor may feel they are doing the patient a favour, but from the patient's viewpoint the doctor is being negligent by passing responsibility to the patient, and even abusing their medical authority to prescribe. A similar incident happened to another respondent, whose reaction is even more critical:

> Have experiences with doctors who on several occasions prescribe medicines that have conflicted with other medicines I usually take. Don't trust the system we have in Sweden when it comes to supervision of patients' drug use.

For this respondent, every time a doctor prescribes a medicine with the potential for an adverse drug interaction, his trust in doctors, even the Swedish healthcare system, is further reduced. As seen, a prescription materializes authority and expertise on the doctors' part, but also trust on the patients' part. Aware of the intrinsic institutional hierarchy and knowledge gap in any medical consultation, people approach doctors for their expertise and expect a certain quality of care. When prescribing is neither professional nor attentive, the quality and accountability of the service, together with the prescriptions, may arouse suspicion: the value of the official healthcare service will be reconsidered, and people may turn to alternative service providers. Individual freedom and liberal market logic are advocated across Swedish society. Paternalism, embedded in the once relatively solid doctor–patient relationship, no longer determines how people process medical knowledge or conform to expertise, nor does it mandate how people should obtain their medicines. When healthcare services are increasingly digitalized, how then do people relate to institutional legitimacy on the Internet?

The logo

Turning from offline encounters to the online setting, our analysis starts with a logo. According to the annual report by the Swedish Pharmacy Association (2018), online retail sales by Swedish pharmacies increased from SEK 80 million a month in 2015 to SEK 250

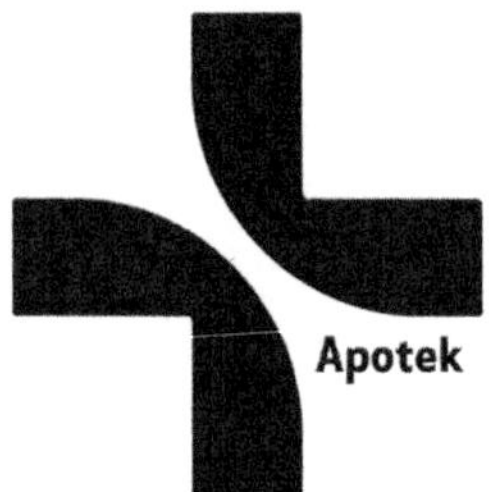

Figure 9.1.

million a month by the end of 2017. In 2017, e-commerce accounted for over 90 per cent of the volume growth. To regulate the online pharmaceutical market, the European Commission launched a logo (Figure 9.1) in 2014, representing the authorization of online pharmacies. All online pharmacies that operate legally in EU must display the logo on their homepage, and that includes the authorized Swedish pharmacies. Yet little empirical data is available regarding its effectiveness among the public (Sugiura 2018).

Two-thirds of respondents in our survey did not recognize the logo, which echoes what the Swedish Medical Products Agency (MPA) (2015) reported. Nearly half of our respondents do not feel safe purchasing medicines online. In response to whether the EU logo would matter when shopping online for medicine, attitudes range from full support to total negation. Some respondents believe having a logo like this would ensure the quality of medicines sold in online pharmacies, 'especially after the deregulation of the pharmaceutical market, it is important to know one is shopping in a real pharmacy'. But this logo alone does not seem persuasive enough for many respondents, because 'it is possible to have this logo without being a real pharmacy. Together with other quality measures it would feel more legitimate'. At the other end of the scale, there was strong scepticism. The logo does not seem accountable because 'it feels too easy to plagiarize and misuse logos on the Internet'. In between the two opposite attitudes, some respondents reacted with varying degrees of uncertainty, still planning to do some sort of quality control on online pharmacies, but doubting whether the EU's logo counts as useful validation. Agency is manifested in different strategies to discern which medicines might be safe to be consumed, such as checking 'if it is the same active ingredients' or looking for 'something on that website that I feel is reliable'.

Given the various responses, we would argue that the assumed association between the EU logo and authorization of online pharmacies is problematic. The logo was introduced with a clear political intention of flagging medicine quality and legal business operations, the assumption being that it would assist consumers in telling reliable online pharmacies apart from rogue ones. However, whether an online logo like this will be deemed valid hinges on other factors. For example, as one respondent explicitly stated, 'If I bought medicine online and needed it cheap and fast, I would probably buy from the first website that offers it'. Further, despite some respondents embracing this top-down political initiative, the suspicion and resistance of many others is worth particular attention. In a dematerialized digital environment, the absence of tangibility or corporeality can lead to higher levels of uncertainty and perceived risk (Bardhi & Eckhardt 2017), in contrast to the traditional form of medical consultation, which is often charac-terized as material, embodied, and sensual (Lupton 1997, 2018). In this scenario, the accumulation of trust in products or services rapidly dissipates, even as the consumer remains fully dependent on recognizing individual objects visualized on a flat computer screen. Our respondents, who in other respects have crafted at least some skills in everyday digital consumption, find it difficult to accept the logo's institutional legitimacy. This also suggests that respondents form a multifaceted knowledge repertoire, which amounts to a knowledge network. Its scale extends beyond the con-sumption of medicines to tie into a much larger setting—everyday consumption praxis. Market offerings, including the logo, are not taken passively. Instead, their value, and especially their practical benefit, is carefully reflected on by transferring information and skills learned from other consumption practices to the activity of online medicine shopping.

Although the authorities frame the act of shopping for medicines outside the legal market as risky and deviant (Sugiura 2018), respondents present themselves as digital consumers—indeed, as craft digital consumers (Campbell 2005)—capable of identifying the pitfalls in the virtual market. Whereas in liberal market thinking this skill is desirable as it produces empowered individuals, one side effect appears to be an ephemeral, fluid attachment to authority. People are increasingly expected to take care of their own health; failing to do so may lead to downgraded healthcare, and even a denial of access to welfare services in general (Michailakis & Schirmer 2010). Self-care is associated with strong morality, as responsibility falls on individuals to not just make a choice, but to make a right choice to perform the duty of good citizens (Alftberg & Hansson 2012). Yet as virtual platforms lift the restrictions on the provision of and access to medicines, it to some extent raises the bar to manifest individual responsibility in a more flexible and reflexive manner. We have previously found that many people believe the level of self-care should be measured against whether one should be prioritized to receive care (Funestrand et al. 2019; Lundin 2008). This is the backdrop to our respondents demonstrating complex attitudes towards the EU logo or liberal virtual markets. Although respondents claim that some kind of quality certification of online pharmacies is needed, the authority embodied by this specific logo seems limited, even invalidated. In other words, the effect of the logo's assumed empowerment is countered by the enactment of individual agency, which enables people to 'express themselves in ways that reify their individualism' (Comor 2011, 322).

Some respondents simply dismiss this way of buying medicine alternative out of hand. Neither supportive nor critical, they claim they would only shop in the bricks-and-mortar pharmacies, so they 'don't feel the need to check the authorization' and the online authorization mark does not speak to them either. To understand this, we draw on the analytical concept of refusal. Refusal is rarely performed in the same way as resistance, nor does it have to involve active non-conformity or strong criticism (Weiss 2016). Rather than focusing on structural reforms, refusers may put an emphasis on the 'health and vitality of immediate social relations' (Sobo 2016, 343). It is evident that our respondents are well aware of the online alternative, but some choose to ignore or stay away from it. As a social act, refusal in the form of avoidance can thus be seen as privileging certain social relations over others (Sobo 2016). The respondents who refuse to shop for medicines online, regardless of logos and other types of quality control, choose to vest their trust in the more solid relations with physical pharmacies and more personal interactions. They also appear reluctant to transfer their established trust from physical pharmacies to digital shopping channels that seem dematerialized and less personal. Here refusal can be conceptualized as an exercise in individual agency, designed to reduce risk by attributing authority to specific information channels. While agency is shaped and enabled by processes and structures, it also co-evolves with consumption practices (Fuentes & Sörum 2019). In the act of refusal, rather than just rebuffing new consumption alternatives, people intentionally disenable authority by shunning it. It is difficult to tell from the survey data exactly which worries discouraged the respondents from buying medicine online, but we can still conclude that respondents used their knowledge networks to make what they believe are sensible choices when it comes to shopping for medicines. Under the surface of quiet abstention (Weiss 2016), agency is practiced as a no to liquid social relations, but a yes to individual responsibility.

Is there a cure out there?

To capture the point at which respondents would consider leaving formal healthcare, we asked them in which situations they would consider buying medicines or treatments that are neither legal in Sweden nor scientifically proved. Most respondents comment that this is a difficult question, as they have never encountered such situations. However, the act of formulating an answer and imagining a breaking point where they would move away from the legal zone uncovers any ambivalent feelings towards biotechnology.

There is consensus among respondents that being affected by a detrimental disease leaves people desperate. It therefore is understandable that they will try every possible treatment, because if 'one has a serious disease, one would be willing to do everything to become healthy again'. Here, the underlying message is that a healthy life is the norm that every person should aim for. In Swedish society, people are increasingly expected to live up to the ideal of having a healthy lifestyle (Michailakis & Schirmer 2010), which somehow legitimizes the hunt for a cure. Further, as we have argued in earlier studies on the cultural meaning of biotechnology, the notion of health is elastic, because modern technologies are ascribed an enormous potential to heal and strengthen the body—'Old truths about nature's inflexibility are replaced by an understanding of its changeability' (Lundin 2002, 339). Rather than being a solid form of existence, the body is increasingly conceptualized as an atomized object, modified to adapt to ever-emerging cultural ideals. Medicines then become one of the desired-for tools with which to calibrate the body to those ideals. National borders, coinciding with the legal boundaries, may give a sense of safety, signalling the quality assurance of the Swedish national health service. However, when 'doctors say no more alternatives are available', or when 'one doesn't get help but is tossed back and forth like a ball', many respondents consider this a legitimate reason to step outside the system and turn to the extra-legal market. This transition is not without its hesitations. It takes time, energy, bravery, and knowledge to deal with the dilemmas and uncertainties, and ultimately the optimism of envisaging a healthy life.

> I think some medicines are illegal for a reason, so I would only do that in desperation, if I didn't have other choices. In this case I would study the medicines as well as I can before I bought and used them.

Desperation is highlighted in many comments. When health professionals announce the end of a search for cures and decide to withdraw treatment, the search for the patients' part is far from over. To be desperate in no way equates to hopelessness or irrational choices; on the contrary, as the quote shows, it implies a determination to find the cure in a strategic manner, such as by studying the medicines very carefully. What can also be taken from this quote is a reluctance to leave formal healthcare for a market of unknown medicines. Medical expertise is still much needed and appreciated by the majority of laypeople, whose medical knowledge is rather limited, especially when their health is deteriorating. Even so, when all the possibilities of formal healthcare are exhausted, it leaves individuals little choice but to feel obliged to take responsibility on their own. In the dispersed, multidimensional knowledge network we conceptualized earlier, 'authority is no longer an alternative to doubt' (Giddens 1991, 195). This differs from the paternalistic doctor–patient relationship where doctors possess the authoritative power of giving orders to patients. Faced with serious diseases where no treatment or medicines are legally available, patients experience dependence on medical authority just as much as doubt towards it. The hunt for a cure continues, although reluctance persists.

Sometimes what holds together the search for a cure is a belief in medical pluralism. It is mediated through the increased mobility of people, goods and information across national boundaries.

> Absolutely! I think there are different ways to look at medication in other countries and it's not to be underestimated in serious situations. What we have in Sweden feels safe and (scientifically) proved, but not in the forefront. If I were diagnosed with a disease with no treatment in Sweden, I would look for alternatives on the Internet and abroad.

It is obvious that this respondent conceives of a boundary, or more specifically limitations on the Swedish national healthcare system. She also exhibits an awareness of alternative medical systems in other countries. Lack of legally available treatments in one system is not the end of the story, since cures might be found in other places where medical approaches are more aggressive or inclusive. Lay understanding of medicines may be insufficient, but identifying where and how to source information is already a crafted skill for many individuals. Further, clearly put by one respondent and echoed by many others, medicines and treatments that are illegitimate in Sweden 'may actually be legally approved or scientifically established in other countries'. This view points at a blurred line between legality and illegality. It also illustrates an adaptive, fluid interpretation of medical knowledge.

'Try googling various healing properties of cannabis. You may start wondering why it is forbidden', a respondent suggests, a confusion arising from a mismatch in information on the Internet and from medical authorities. One can choose to follow the advice of medical professionals who do not have much to offer at the moment, while out there, somewhere in the extra-legal market, there seems to be hope (see Brown & Michael 2003; for hope, see also Idvall in this volume). Who to believe and how to choose? At this crossroads many people, including but certainly not limited to our respondents, cast about for a moral standpoint, between taking individual responsibility on the one hand and assuming the role of ethical citizen-consumer on the other. In searching for a possible cure, national borders and the laws that define them are contested. More tellingly, it enables individuals to justify their transgressions without feeling morally wrong. This is the point at which the legally grey market is transformed into a moral market, which lessens the paradox of exercising individual agency without neglecting the duty of being a righteous citizen.

Whereas some respondents say they would be perfectly willing to grasp at straws, many adopt a calculating mindset, weighing up the worth of buying medicines illicitly. 'There must be something that really convinces me that it's worth trying', says a respondent. Whether the treatment will outweigh its side effects; whether the medicine comes from a country one can trust; whether one can financially afford such a medical solution: all these uncertainties are pondered over by respondents. Between the lines of the imagined presuppositions, their resistance reveals how tempting it is to shift the moral boundaries. What is more, technological advancements pave the way for it. To some extent, technologies are evocative objects (Turkle 2011). Many respondents are positive towards technological innovations, but are caught in the dilemma of choosing between doctors and markets. Worth here seems to be a question with a mathematical answer, but much more than that: many uncertainties might worsen the present situation, yet that risk is balanced by a strong desire to live what is perceived as a normal, healthy life. Far from a simple calculation of pros and cons, this is also about now and then. As one respondent says, 'Now I would never consider doing so, but if I were dying?'. With a future full of uncertainties, risk-taking is an essential and inescapable aspect of everyday life (Giddens 1991). What is left to leverage the final decision of leaving, or not, for the extra-legal market, is perhaps how much faith one has in biotechnologies, and how much confidence one can afford to live with a disease. These are variables on a spectrum, engineering a variety of social realities which are then materialized as different consumption strategies. As a result, the value of medical products and healthcare services becomes fragile, particularly when doctors' sole authority, together with their medical knowledge, is faced with competition.

Nonetheless, before making for the grey zone, one respondent leaves a final remark.

> Doctors nowadays are constrained by rules and do not dare to seek in a scientific way for new knowledge; but often resign themselves (in my experience in recent years) to diagnosing and prescribing medicines. If the diagnosis can't be made, the activity = zero and the answer is just Oh well... Oh yeah. That means there are gaps in the medics' role in constantly improving medicine.

There is a hope here, or rather an expectation, that doctors will take the lead. For many laypeople, doctors still play an important role in their healthcare. And people are willing to invest in a functioning doctor–patient relationship (see Brown & Michael 2003). Following instructions on what to do and what not is regarded as obstructing doctors from fully utilizing their expertise and medical knowledge. Doctors' inflexibility, as our respondents experience it, their refusal to step outside the safety zone, makes doctor–patient collaborations difficult. Furthermore, as skilled prosumers, our respondents claim equal power relationships with doctors—but while attempting to fit into the role of responsible citizens. The notion of taking care of one's own body, however, does not indicate a dramatic overturning of the power hierarchy. In a society where medical knowledge, products, and services are far more accessible through multiple channels than ever before, marketplaces outside the official healthcare system appear more attractive to laypeople (see Hansson, Nilsson & Tiberg in this volume). One explanation might be that such marketplaces signal their potential to meet people's basic needs for medical care. Perhaps more importantly, though, the grey zones in the market offer people tangible tools with which to conform to the image of an ethical, healthy citizen-consumer (Kristensen et al. 2016).

Becoming a health agent

In a society saturated with digital products and services, with a strong emphasis on individual responsibility, and instilled with political strategies to introduce market logic to the public sector, seeking healthcare and medication takes on new forms. The Internet is transforming how the pharmaceutical market is organized and how knowledge moves (Sugiura 2018). This is seen in many societies with neoliberal politics, and not least in Sweden from where our empirical material is taken.

In considering the empirical problem of the widespread availability of SF medical products and the increasing number of people buying medicines illegitimately, we examine both the online and offline scenarios which may lead to the purchase of medicines in extra-legal markets. One observation is the emergence of a network where knowledge from a variety of sources is collected and synthesized, produced and consumed. Rather than being confined to a healthcare context, we find that this network also expands and becomes entangled with daily consumption praxis. It enables knowledge to flow seamlessly from one context to another. Many respondents are well aware of the risks of removing themselves from formal healthcare, and this explains why many of them feel dependent on medical professionals' expertise to access the right medicines. But simultaneously, they maintain their right to doubt authority. This implies that the reliance on medical authority should be interpreted differently from that in the traditional, paternalistic doctor–patient relationship. As authority no longer comes from a single source, knowledge can be understood as constructed using diverse channels. Although knowledge possessed by medical professionals is still deemed important, it increasingly becomes part of a 'personalized repertoire' (Kristensen et al. 2016, 496). There is a pattern to our findings, where respondents prosume knowledge and craft their skills before they decide which medicines to buy and where. In this prosumption process, individual agency is performed in various ways: by equipping oneself with necessary medical knowledge, by doubting medical diagnoses, or even by refusing to use authorized online pharmacies. All these suggest an ephemeral or loosening attachment to the authorities and their expertise.

While laypeople may have turned themselves into skilled prosumers—active, empowered, free agents, making choices according to a market logic—they may also risk becoming 'an agent of increasingly complex forms of possessive individualism' (Comor 2011, 322), only entrenching the status quo. As studies of the phenomenon of medical travel remind us, agency and victimhood constitute one another. People who seek organ transplants, fertility treatments, or stem cell treatments in the grey markets or even black markets are actually driven by a desire to conform to normalized images. These images—having a healthy body or accomplishing parenthood—are imposed by society on individuals (for example, Humbracht et al. 2016; Lundin 2015; Pande 2014). These deeply rooted normalities in sociocultural structures enact agency in those people who are commonly considered as victims. Our study of illegitimate medicine purchases aligns with this argument; it is especially apparent when respondents are asked to consider when they would leave formal healthcare. Our findings further demonstrate that victimhood also inherently resides in the enactment of agency. Becoming prosumers, people are tasked with anchoring themselves with a moral standpoint to fit with the constantly shifting imagery of a healthy body. However, as our respondents said, at times they experience the formal healthcare system as inflexible and bureaucratic. It is not surprising, then, that people begin to oscillate between institutions and markets, in search of an authoritative and trusted voice.

Care, after all, is a collaborative practice (Mol 2008). Even in a society that endorses the rise of consumerism, advocates individual empowerment, and is increasingly informed by market thinking, a balanced doctor–patient relationship is still much desired among respondents. However, this particular service encounter has to be a relational one that allows for different degrees of dependence as well as the negotiation of power (Trnka & Trundle 2014). To do so, we have to acknowledge the multistability of knowledge production. Applied to the phenomenon of SF medical products, failing to perceive knowledge in its multifaceted forms may lead prosumers to seek healthcare and medication elsewhere, even outside the formal public health system. A legal grey market then comes into sight where low-quality medicines can circulate and cause harm.

Notes

1 All quotes in this chapter are taken from our study 'Where and how do you buy medicine', part of the research project 'Illegal drugs: Gathering information from the public and doctors: A preliminary evaluation of the implementation of knowledge in society', supported by the Erik Philip Sorensen Foundation 2017 (H2016-015)

and VINNOVA (VLU14-1006, V16-0307). Another part of the research was focused on physicians' attitudes towards a liberal pharmaceutical market and evolving consumption patterns in Sweden (see Funestrand et al. 2019).

2 Digital care has grown dramatically in Sweden after we conducted our study, and a growing number of people are turning to e-doctors (Ekman et al. 2019).

References

Alfadl, Abubakr, Mohamed Hassali & Mohamed Izham Ibrahim (2013), 'Counterfeit drug demand: Perceptions of policymakers and community pharmacists in Sudan', *Research in Social & Administrative Pharmacy*, 9(3), 310–19.

Alftberg, Åsa & Kristofer Hansson (2012), 'Introduction: Self-care translated into practice', *Culture Unbound: Journal of Current Cultural Research*, 4, 415–24.

Attaran, Amir (2015), 'Stopping murder by medicine: Introducing the Model Law on medicine crime', *American Journal of Tropical Medicine & Hygiene*, 92(6), 127–32.

Bardhi, Fleura & Giana Eckhardt (2017), 'Liquid consumption', *Journal of Consumer Research*, 44(3), 582–97.

Bauman, Zygmunt (2000), *Liquid modernity* (Cambridge: Polity).

Bloom, Gerald, Hilary Standing & Robert Lloyd (2008), 'Markets, information asymmetry and health care: Towards new social contracts', *Social Science & Medicine*, 66(10), 2076–87.

Brissman, Gustav (2016), 'Illegala och förfalskade läkemedel i Sverige: En etnografisk studie av svenskars attityder till att handla läkemedel illegalt' (unpub. report, Lund: Lunds universitet).

Brown, Nik & Mike Michael (2003), 'A sociology of expectations: Retrospecting prospects and prospecting retrospects', *Technology Analysis & Strategic Management*, 15(1), 3–18.

Campbell, Colin (2005), 'The craft consumer: Culture, craft and consumption in a postmodern society', *Journal of Consumer Culture*, 5(1), 23–42.

Clark, Fiona (2015), 'Rise in online pharmacies sees counterfeit drugs go global', *The Lancet*, 386(10001), 1327–8.

Comor, Edward (2011), 'Contextualizing and critiquing the fantastic prosumer: Power, alienation and hegemony', *Critical Sociology*, 37(3), 309–327.

Ekman, Björn, Hans Thulesius, Jens Wilkens, Ana Lindgren, Olof Cronberg & Eva Arvidsson (2019), 'Utilization of digital primary care in Sweden: Descriptive analysis of claims data on demographics, socioeconomics, and diagnoses', *International Journal of Medical Informatics*, 127, 134–40.

Fuentes, Christian & Niklas Sörum (2019), 'Agencing ethical consumers: Smartphone apps and the socio-material reconfiguration of everyday life', *Consumption Markets & Culture*, 22(2), 131–56.

Funestrand, Henrik, Rui Liu, Susanne Lundin & Margareta Troein (2019), 'Substandard and falsified medical products are a global public health threat: A pilot survey of awareness among physicians in Sweden', *Journal of Public Health*, 41(1), e95-e102.

Giddens, Anthony (1991), *Modernity and self-identity: Self and society in the late modern age* (Cambridge: Polity).

Gunnarson, Martin & Susanne Lundin (2015), 'The complexities of victimhood: Insights from the organ trade', *Somatechnics*, 5(1), 32–51.

Hall, Alexandra & Georgios Antonopoulos (2016), *Fake meds online: The internet and the transnational market in illicit pharmaceuticals* (Basingstoke: Palgrave Macmillan).

Hornberger, Julia & Erma Cossa (2012), *From drug safety to drug security: The policing of counterfeit medications* (Johannesburg: African Centre for Migration & Society).

Humbracht, Michael, Insoo Hyun & Susanne Lundin (2016), 'Managing hope and spiritual distress: The centrality of the doctor–patient relationship in combatting stem cell travel', in Erik Malmkvist & Kristin Zeiler (eds.), *Bodily exchanges, bioethics and border crossing: Perspectives on giving, selling and sharing bodies* (Abingdon: Routledge).

Kristensen, Dorthe Brogård, Ming Lim & Søren Askegaard (2016), 'Healthism in Denmark: State, market, and the search for a "Moral Compass"', *Health: An Interdisciplinary Journal for the Social Study of Health, Illness & Medicine*, 20(5), 485–504.

Liang, Bryan & Tim Mackey (2012), 'Sexual medicine: Online risks to health—The problem of counterfeit drugs', *Nature Reviews Urology*, 9(9), 482–3.

Liu, Rui & Susanne Lundin (2016), 'Falsified medicines: Literature review', *Working Papers in Medical Humanities*, 2(1), 1–25.

Lock, Margaret & Vinh-Kim Nguyen (2010), *An anthropology of biomedicine* (Chichester: Wiley-Blackwell).

Lundin, Susanne (2002), 'Creating identity with biotechnology: The xenotransplanted body as the norm', *Public Understanding of Science*, 11(4), 333–45.

—— (2008), 'Old bodies—new technologies', *Ethnologie Française*, 38(2), 277–81.

—— (2015), *Organs for sale: An ethnographic examination of the international organ trade* (Houndmills: Palgrave Macmillan).

Lupton, Deborah (1997), 'Consumerism, reflexivity and the medical encounter', *Social Science & Medicine*, 45(3), 373–81.

—— (2018), *Digital health: Critical and cross-disciplinary perspectives* (Abingdon: Routledge).

Michailakis, Dimitris & Werner Schirmer (2010), 'Agents of their health? How the Swedish welfare state introduces expectations of individual responsibility', *Sociology of Health & Illness*, 32(6), 930–47.

Mol, Annemarie (2002), *The body multiple: Ontology in medical practice* (Durham: Duke University Press).

—— (2008), *The logic of care: Health and the problem of patient choice* (Abingdon: Routledge).

Nayyar, Gaurvika, Joel Breman, Tim Mackey, John Clark, Mustapha Hajjou, Megan Littrell & James Herrington (2019), 'Falsified and Substandard Drugs: Stopping the Pandemic', *American Journal of Tropical Medicine & Hygiene*, 100(5), 1058–65.

Newton, Paul, Céline Caillet & Philippe Guerin (2016), 'A link between poor quality antimalarials and malaria drug resistance?', *Expert Review of Anti-Infective Therapy*, 14(6), 531–3.

Nordstrom, Carolyn (2007), *Global outlaws: Crime, money, and power in the contemporary world* (Berkeley & Los Angeles: University of California Press).

Pande, Amrita (2014), *Wombs in labor: Transnational commercial surrogacy in India* (New York: Columbia University).

Rebiere, Hérve, Pauline Guinot, Denis Chauvey & Charlotte Brenier (2017), 'Fighting falsified medicines: The analytical approach', *Journal of Pharmaceutical & Biomedical Analysis*, 142, 286–306.

Ritzer, George (2015), 'The "new" world of prosumption: Evolution, "return of the same," or revolution?', *Sociological Forum*, 30(1), 1–17.

Sobo, Elisa (2016), 'Theorizing (vaccine) refusal: Through the looking glass', *Cultural Anthropology (Society for Cultural Anthropology)*, 31(3), 342–50.

Sugiura, Lisa (2018), *Respectable deviance and purchasing medicine online: Opportunities and risks for consumers* (Cham: Springer International).

Sugiura, Lisa, Catherine Pope & Craig Webber (2012), 'Buying unlicensed slimming drugs from the web: A virtual ethnography', in *Proceedings of the 4th Annual ACM Web Science Conference (WebSci '12)* (New York: Association for Computing Machinery).

Swedish Medical Products Agency (2015), *Köp av receptbelagda läkemedel från osäkra källor på internet* (Uppsala: Läkemedelsverket), https://lakemedelsverket.se/upload/om-lakemedelsverket/rapporter/Rapport-Kop-av-receptbelagda-lakeme-del-fran-osakra-kallor-pa-internet-enkatundersokning-plus-bilaga-2015.pdf

Swedish Pharmacy Association (2018), *Branschrapport 2018* (Stockholm: Sveriges Apoteksförening Service), http://www.sverigesapoteksforening.se/branschrapport-2018/.

Trnka, Susanne & Catherine Trundle (2014), 'Competing responsibilities: Moving beyond neoliberal responsibilisation', *Anthropological Forum*, 24(2), 136–53.

Turkle, Sherry (2011), *Evocative objects: Things we think with* (Cambridge, MA: MIT Press).

Weiss, Erica (2016), 'Refusal as act, refusal as abstention', *Cultural Anthropology*, 31(3), 351–8.

Whyte, Susan, Sjaak van der Geest & Anita Hardon (2002), *Social lives of medicines* (Cambridge: CUP).

WHO (2017), *Global surveillance and monitoring system for substandard and falsified medical products* (Geneva: WHO).

List of abbreviations

CRISPR	clustered regularly interspaced short palindromic repeats, a family of DNA sequences
FUB	Swedish National Association for People with Intellectual Disability
GRC	Guidelines Review Committee
HCK	Swedish Disability Federation Central Committee
IBFAN	International Baby Food Action Network
MPA	Medical Products Agency
NCD	non-communicable disease
NGO	non-governmental organization
OTC	over-the-counter
POM	prescription-only medicines
RCT	randomized controlled trials
RFSU	Swedish Association for Sexuality Education
SEK	Swedish kronor
SF	substandard and falsified
STS	science and technology studies
UN	United Nations
UNICEF	United Nations Children's Fund
WHA	World Health Assembly
WHO	World Health Organization

About the authors

Åsa Alftberg, PhD in Ethnology, is a lecturer at the Department of Social Work, Malmö University. Her research concerns the body and health, in particular ageing and eldercare. Other research interests are the implementation and circulation of medical knowledge.

Kristofer Hansson is a lecturer at the Department of Social Work, Malmö University and holds an Associate Professorship in Ethnology. His research focuses on children and young people living with long-term sickness and disability, as well as medical praxis in health care and emerging new biomedical technologies.

Markus Idvall is Associate Professor in Ethnology at the Department of Ethnology, History of Religion and Gender Studies, Stockholm University. In a current research project he focuses on medical aspects of the reception of refugees and border control in Sweden at the end of the Second World War and beyond.

Rachel Irwin is a researcher at the Department of Arts and Cultural Sciences, Lund University. She has a PhD in social anthropology from the London School of Hygiene and Tropical Medicine. Her research interests are the formation of global health policies, the history of Swedish development aid, and global health engagement.

Max Liljefors is Professor of Art History and Visual Studies at the Department of Arts and Cultural Sciences, Lund University, and Visiting Professor of Media Aesthetics at the University of Bergen. He has published extensively on performance, body, and video art, the visual cultures of the biosciences, and visual historiography.

His current research concerns aesthetic theory, art and religion, and arts and health.

Karolina Lindh, PhD in Information Studies, is a librarian at the Faculty of Medicine at Lund University. Her research focuses on how standardized knowledge is configured in health practices and how biomedicine is communicated to the public.

Rui Liu, MA in Applied Cultural Analysis, is a postgraduate research student at the Department of Service Management and Service Studies, Campus Helsingborg, Lund University. Her research interests lie in the emergence of grey pharmaceutical markets, evolving health consumption strategies, and the production of health knowledge.

Susanne Lundin is Professor of Ethnology at the Department of Arts and Cultural Sciences, Lund University, and affiliated to Stellenbosch Institute of Advanced Study (STIAS), Wallenberg Research Centre at Stellenbosch University. She has published widely on the body in health and illness, medical technologies, and social change. Her research interests in recent years concern medical treatments, and medicines in the global black market.

Gabriella Nilsson is Associate Professor in Ethnology at the Department of Arts and Cultural Sciences, Lund University. Her research focus is how power is done, both structurally and individually, and specifically in relation to gender and violence, child health, work, and ageing.

Irén Tiberg, PhD in Nursing, of the Department of Health Sciences, Medical Faculty at Lund University. She has a long clinical background as a paediatric nurse, specialized in paediatric diabetes. Her research focuses on children and adolescents with long-term illnesses such as type 1 diabetes, and involves the development, evaluation, and implementation of interventions related to health-care organization and e-health.

Anna Tunlid is Associate Professor in the History of Ideas and Sciences at Lund University. Her research focuses on the history of life sciences and medicine, and especially the history of genetics. A particular focus has been the relation between the development of knowledge and various societal and political interests.